FIRE YOUR DOCTOR

CHOOSE LIFE

by

Paul Keenan

ISBN-13: 978-1976479984

ISBN-10: 1976479983

www.antarana.com

paulkeenan@antarana.com

Reviews

Important Notice

The information in this book is presented for the educational and free exchange of ideas and speech in relation to health and wellness only. It is not intended to diagnose any physical or mental condition, or to prescribe or promote any particular product(s). It is not intended as a substitute for the advice and treatment of a licensed professional. In the event you use any information within the book for your own health, you are prescribing for yourself, which is your constitutional right and for which the author of this book assumes no responsibility.

Foreword

What can we do in an Age where serious disease is at frightening proportions and medical doctors will not or cannot cure? When their interventions make us worse, not better? When Alternatives do not work for us, either?

When years of modern medicine proved ineffective, in resolving physical and mental disorders, Paul Keenan turned to alternatives. Over two decades there was hardly a therapy he did not try. Frustrated by the inability of modern and alternative medicine to cure him and close to breakdown, Paul was left with no choice. He **FIRED HIS DOCTORS**, fleeing abroad, in a desperate attempt to save his sanity and recover his health.

When, in an Indian backwater, a traditional Ayurvedic healer reversed his arthritis, Paul's eyes were opened to the power of natural healing. Inspired by this experience, Paul spent the following years studying the methods of the great healing masters, learning what makes us sick and what we need to get well.

Fire Your Doctor Choose Life presents, in plain language, the latest research, forgotten knowledge, common sense and simple methods of healing, to offer new hope.

Dedication

This book is dedicated to my dear mother, who did not deserve to suffer as she did. If she were still here, I would wrap her in my arms and apologize for my lack of understanding of just how sick she was. Instead, I have written this book to honour her memory and the memory of untold millions like her who, desperately needing cures, died disappointed.

I also dedicate this book to my children, Michael, Lauren and Neil, who wanted their father to be a hero, only to find he was mortal.

Finally, I dedicate this book to YOU. The courageous person, seeking to reverse disease, who knows, instinctively, nature holds the key.

Acknowledgments

I acknowledge the champions of the last century, who fought to bring important healing knowledge to the world. Dr John Christopher; Dr Max Gerson and his daughter Charlotte; Dr Richard Schulze; Linus Pauling; Dr Abram Hoffer; Gandhi, who established 'Nature Cure' Centres throughout India, and the traditional Ayurvedic healers I met, who with compassion, devotion and skill, showed me a better way.

Special mention to Chris Woollams, founder of the 'CancerActive' charity and author of several books, including 'Everything You Need to Know to Help You Beat Cancer', whose prompting led me to write this book.

Who Should Buy This Book?

Everyone! At the rates of sickness we are seeing, you are virtually guaranteed to succumb to one or more chronic, degenerative, disorders by the time you are 50.

Cancer
Heart Disease
Diabetes
Arthritis
Obesity
Anxiety, Depression, Bipolar, ADHD, Addiction
Fibromyalgia
Hypertension
Allergies
Alzheimer's
Asthma
Chronic Fatigue Syndrome
AIDS
Gastrointestinal Diseases – Crohn's, Colitis, Diverticulitis, IBS
Metabolic Disorder
Autoimmune Disorders –MS, Celiac Disease, RA
Many others!

"You know you suffered many years with physical and psychological disorders?" prodded the Naturopath.

"Yes", I responded.

"And you know you travelled the world looking for cures?"

"Uh-huh", I replied, wondering where this was heading.

"I could have cured you in three days".

TABLE OF CONTENTS

DAN

84 year old Canadian, Dan, was a gentle giant. When he came shuffling up my drive, he couldn't bend his fingers, they were so swollen with Rheumatoid Arthritis. Dan was 40kg overweight and understandably down in the dumps. A big meat-eater all his life he told me about his triple heart-bypass, cancer and how the medications he was taking only made his Arthritis worse. Dan had certainly experienced his share of illness.

"I am too old", he said. *"The Doctors have written me off"*.

Alternative practitioners refused to help Dan because he was high risk. They do not have the protection of the State and could go to jail if Dan suddenly dropped dead on their doorstep. I explained that, for the same reasons, I could not help.

"Please", said Dan. *"Nobody else will help me"*.

My heart went out to this dignified man so I recommended a simple program with a track record of safety and success. Dan came off most of his medications and commenced a citrus-based, juice fast. Like most people Dan could not imagine going two hours without eating but nevertheless committed to the program.

After 7 days, Dan was feeling so well he asked to do 3 days more. After 10, he called again and said he was feeling even better and could he continue? I suggested he stop at 14.

On the morning of the 15th day, Dan walked up my drive, transformed. He had lost 9kgs, looked ten years younger, his arthritis symptoms were gone and his depression had lifted. It was wonderful to see.

"How did you get on with the juices?" I asked.

"It was easy after the first day", said Dan. *"I wish I could have continued"*.

Introduction

"You're FIRED!"

More of us should try it, don't you think? Walk into our Doctor's office, look them in the eye and give it to them straight.

If you think about it, the idea you would buy a book titled **'Fire Your Doctor'** is an act of independence and defiance some might consider revolutionary. I am sure you were not thinking that when you picked this off the bookshelf or ordered it online. You just want to know how to fix your Arthritis or Cancer or Diabetes or Allergies.

Welcome to the 'Bypass Age'. An Age, where, if Doctors cannot or will not cure you, you bypass them. An Age where, if drug corporations, Medical Associations, 'captured' Consumer Protection Agencies and 'revolving-door' government flunkies erect barriers to change, you bypass them, too. Around 50% of patients are using Complementary and Alternative Medicine (CAM), bypassing their Doctors.

A revolution in Health Care is certainly needed. We are the sickest species on the planet and getting sicker. Mankind cannot sustain this expensive, technological-chemical assault on our bodies, minds and environment, for much longer. The number of us succumbing to chronic, degenerative disorders is too great. Perhaps it will come when 1 in 2 of our children is Autistic (as projected). Perhaps it will come when more than half of us die from Cancer (we are nearly there now). When corporations make more money CURING disease than TREATING it. Or, as a Doctor friend bluntly put it,

"When the owners and CEOs of 'Big Food', 'Big Pharma' and the vaccine makers are all swinging from the same branch."

It is coming. I hear it with every phone call and from every visitor I receive. They may use different words but the message is the same.

"I am sick and my Doctor cannot cure me."

An explosion of interest in Natural and Alternative methods of healing is happening and you and I are part of it. Quite when we reach tipping point, where wholesale change will come, is hard to say. It isn't just Health Care that needs to change. Doctors are those we see AFTER we have fallen ill. What is making us sick BEFORE we see the Doctor also needs to change. The choices you and I make, every single day, consciously or unconsciously, that build health or build disease. Think about that. **Every choice you make is either building health or building**

disease. Are you fully conscious of this? Or is your health 'the Doctor's job' and you don't think about it?

You may not realize it but you are part of a massive shift in human awareness. For the first time in the history of mankind we have access to knowledge the rich and powerful traditionally held. Instant access to more information, in one hour on the internet, than we had in a lifetime, 100 years ago. It is a wonderful window of opportunity which, unfortunately, is closing, with every keystroke and mouse movement tracked and archived, and internet giants increasing their filtering of what we are allowed to see.

When my mother died a painful and undignified death there was no internet and no hope. You accepted what Doctors told you, without question, because 'The Doctor knows best'. Now we understand this is not true. Doctors know only what they have been taught. They treat, only in a way they are allowed to treat. They know nothing about alternatives, pay lip-service to prevention, and your grandmother knows more about nutrition than they do. Today, thanks to the internet, within minutes of your Doctor declaring your condition 'incurable', putting you on a lifetime regime of colourful pills *(while sniffily extinguishing hope something else can cure you)*, you can be online, discovering simple, safe, healing methods you never knew existed. Whether they work or not I will come to but at least you know of their existence.

When I first started researching Rheumatoid Arthritis (RA), the disease that killed my mother, my knowledge of medicine and the health system was non-existent. I was strong (apart from seasonal hay fever) and didn't think about health at all. You don't when you are young. Sickness is something that happens to other people. Then, after my mother passed away, I came across an article explaining that RA responds well to diet. This was the first time I had heard this. I investigated further. At first, curious, then appalled, finally angry, when I discovered Rheumatoid Arthritis is curable, without NSAIDs, Methotrexate, steroids and gold injections, and my mother need not have suffered the terrible end she did. I wanted to know why Doctors did not know about this, when it came from their own literature? Why dietary therapies were not being applied to RA sufferers in hospitals? Why Doctors did not know about natural methods of healing. Juice and water fasts, raw food diets, hydrotherapy and so on. At Antarana, my Wellness Retreat, I see RA symptoms disappear within 10 days, just through dietary change.

Then I discovered a world I had no idea existed. A world where Doctors are not allowed to suggest alternatives, or deviate from 'Standard Practice', otherwise they can be struck off. A frightening dystopian world, where parents of children with cancer can be jailed, or lose their children to the State if they don't submit them to the violent assault that is chemotherapy, radiation and surgery. Even when their odds of survival from such treatments are virtually zero. A world where the State can kidnap your children for not allowing them to be vaccinated, though they may be healthier than other children, under the invented and false pretext of 'herd immunity'. A world gone mad, where what was once normal and natural *(achieving natural immunity)* is now labelled 'child abuse'. Where pharmaceutical 'Robber Barons' control medicine, for profit. Not Doctors, for health.

I started to dig a little deeper and learned how the health system really works as opposed to how I thought it worked. How it is a business, run by businessmen. And as long as treatments make more money than cures, we will have treatments and no cures. Doctors fight valiantly to save lives... I might have died on two occasions without them... but for chronic and degenerative disorders, 75% of what plagues us, they can do little, only make matters worse.

I learned the system is a failure. That it has been **designed** to fail. Because if it succeeded, it would put itself out of business. I discovered an unofficial history of medicine, instead of the approved version, which shed light on why there were no cures. That, when courageous healers dared to cure the sick, the health cops, on behalf of the medical robbers, would persecute them and suppress knowledge of their methods. Often waiting until the healers had made enough money, for the *'smash and grab'* to be worthwhile. In the suppressed 1953 **Fitzgerald Report** the Chief Investigator did not mince his words...

"Public and private funds have been thrown around like confetti at a country fair to close up and destroy clinics, hospitals, and scientific research laboratories which do not conform to the viewpoint of medical associations."

I found out how promising treatments and natural compounds would never be approved because it takes hundreds of millions of dollars to get them through clinical trials. How natural products cannot be patented. Which means only un-natural molecules are approved, even when **known** to be less effective and harmful. Then I understood. This is a very exclusive Club, into which only the wealthiest corporations are granted access.

There was so much more I did not know. How our present-day health system was created and by which powerful, controlling families. Why fossil-fuel-derived, pharmaceutical 'medicine' came to be so dominant and how chemistry and technology came to trump biology *(you may have noticed lately how biology is making a comeback, with 'Bio'-this and 'Bio'-that)*.

I learned why Cancer treatments have not changed in decades and how cancer charities and pink ribbons are a cynical sham, fleecing the public. They must be, if you think about it. The mandated conventional treatment, for over 60 years, is chemotherapy, radiation and surgery. Or else. Doctors attempting non-mandated methods can be struck off. This being the case, why are Cancer charities nagging the public constantly for donations 'for research'? There has been NO serious investigation into alternatives, at all. Quite the opposite. Cancer charities work **with** medical associations to undermine medical schools, hospitals and practitioners, even when they have ample clinical evidence and customer testimonials, showing natural methods produce better outcomes than existing treatments. When you dig, you discover cancer research is almost always designed to fail.

You learn from people like Ben Goldacre, who wrote '**Bad Pharma**', how rigged studies and manipulated science can be used to sell junk food pyramids, junk flu pandemics, junk remedies and dismiss alternatives. You learn of the immense harm pharma drugs cause and the many side effects your Doctor never informed you of. Or learn from **Nature**, a weekly science journal, how most prescribed drugs do not work for the majority that take them. That only 2%, if that, benefit from taking Statins. Which means **98% are only getting the side effects**.

You discover the top 5 drug companies earn more per year than the whole of Africa. That patients get better ON treatment not BECAUSE of treatment. There was so much to take in. Once I started digging I could not stop. Each shocking new revelation chipping away at my childlike trust and naivety regarding Health Care. Or is that Sickness Care?

I learned I was an entry in an health corporation's balance sheet, generating expected lifetime revenue of $275,000 from medication, for my 'incurable' disease and if, like many patients, I'm taking three or more medicines, what a bonanza that is for owners and shareholders. That, in the last two years of my life, what was left of my assets (including my home) would be pounced on to pay for cancer treatment or heart by-pass operations. A final mugging by the Corporate State as I passed on. I knew it was true, knowing families who have been thrown out of their homes because a parent, or family member, could not afford health insurance. Or even if they could afford it, were denied by a myriad of exclusions.

I have had a taste of medical racketeering. In an emergency visit to a private hospital, in Thailand, due to food poisoning, it was clear all they cared about was my ability to pay. You could argue this is reasonable. However, when they saw I was a foreigner, the fees were jacked up and suddenly I am pressured to take all kinds of tests and procedures and encouraged to stay 'just a few more days' for 'observation'. A euphemism for, 'we haven't finished picking your pocket yet'. After 4 days, I was relieved to escape with the obligatory shopping trolley full of over-priced meds, sadly, minus my appendix. Thailand's Prime Minister is promising to rein in rampant hospital overcharging, after street protests.

All this is depressing and people do not like to hear it but I needed to know. Because, by not knowing, I had stayed far too long in a system happy to keep me sick. Sometimes I wish I had remained ignorant. It is heart-breaking to see millions suffer and die when their diseases are preventable and can be cured. I have to stay positive. Whatever is happening today does not have to be our future. Instead of passive actors, in this real-life drama, we can be revolutionaries. The vanguard of a human wave, taking back control of our health and that of our children. A wave that seeks to give medicine back its soul. A wave saying to Medical Authorities:

"If you aren't going to cure us, step aside, while we cure ourselves".

Thanks to the internet I discovered my disorders were not 'incurable' after all, learned healers existed who had cured cancer and heart disease, arthritis and diabetes, depression and anxiety. Today, the same methods that cured my arthritis, years ago, in India, can easily be found, with a few mouse-clicks. I can order rain-forest herbs, nutritious drinks, design my own healing program, and source everything I need for it, online. I am in the '**Bypass Age**' and, just as water flows around a rock, I can bypass all that has previously failed and cure myself. The good news is, if I can do it, so can you.

Chapter 1
The Health You Deserve

"We all deserve a life of glowing health and vitality, free from pain and sickness. Whether in body, mind or spirit. It is our birthright. To be happy. To be at peace. To enjoy a long, healthy existence on this beautiful planet. To love ourselves, our families and our fellow man. To pass away peacefully in our sleep. Such a life is attainable if we live wisely, in accordance with natural laws."
- Paul Keenan

A host of mental and physical maladies have befallen mankind, like Biblical plagues. Diseases and disorders I never heard of as a child are now 'incurable' epidemics.

The number of conditions is staggering and getting worse. There are around 80 Auto-Immune disorders, 200 types of Arthritis, 200 different Cancers and over 300 Psychiatric disorders. In the U.S., half of men will get Cancer. 1 in 3 women. When I was young, it was 1 in 25. Coronary artery disease is the No.1 killer, yet barely existed before 1900. 1 BILLION people globally – 70% of Americans, 66% of Britons and 63% of Australians are overweight or obese. Obesity rates in Australia are climbing faster than anywhere else in the world. The cost to society, of obesity-linked disease, is staggering.

Modern medicine can be brilliant with 'acute' and 'emergency' care. Yet, for 'chronic' and 'degenerative' disorders such as cancer, heart and cerebrovascular disease (stroke), which cause 75% of deaths, in industrialized nations, it is a colossal failure. Millions are set to be tortured, scarred, mutilated, poisoned and burned by well-meaning but ignorant medical doctors, attempting to relieve suffering, until they are finally rejected and sent home to die. Think I am exaggerating?

In 2013, the **National Cancer Institute** admitted two important cancers, **early stage breast cancer** and **prostate cancer**, were NOT cancers after all but harmless lesions. Over a 30 year period, 1.3 million women were subjected to a combination of mastectomy, lumpectomy, radiation and chemotherapy. Many more had breasts irradiated and were filled with fear and dread. Who knows how many new cancers this created. The same applies to men diagnosed with a form of prostate cancer. Other cancers were identified, too.

"...many lesions detected during breast, prostate, thyroid, lung and other cancer screenings should not be called cancer at all but should instead be reclassified as IDLE conditions, which stands for "indolent lesions of epithelial origin.""

*"...**hundreds of thousands of men and women are undergoing needless and sometimes disfiguring and harmful treatments** for premalignant and cancerous lesions that are so slow growing they are unlikely to ever cause harm"*

This kind of horrific error would never occur with safer, non-toxic, non-invasive alternatives. In the U.S., Dr Dean Ornish has proven his program, to reverse heart disease using diet, stress reduction and exercise, works. Patients can be out of danger within a month. Yet, a friend who recently underwent triple-bypass surgery, believing he was getting 'brand new plumbing', is carrying livid scars on his leg and chest and has to spend a year recovering. He had never heard of Dean Ornish, or his program, nor had his Doctor ever suggested it.

Why? If someone asked me if I prefer 12 months on a healing diet, or a surgeon saw open my chest, rip out a vein from my leg, plunge a knife into my heart, with the possibility I might die on the operating table, I think I might like a crack at the diet. In what way is undergoing major surgery better than a year eating healthy food, exercising and reducing stress, which will put me out of danger, restore ALL of my circulatory system, resolve other disorders I may have and renew my love of life?

My mother spent her last two years suffering what I can only describe as medieval medical cruelty, due to chronic Rheumatoid Arthritis. The Doctors were conscientious and heroic but limited to pain management, which devastated her body more than the disease. What made it worse is **they knew**. Appalled at her suffering, I asked if there was anything else the family could try? The Doctors said "No". After one-too-many trips to intensive care, she was put out of her misery with an overdose of morphine.

What has happened to healing? Where is the effort to cure disease? We are supposed to have a **Health** system not a **Disease Management** system. When you only manage a disease and make no attempt to address its underlying cause, are you even a Doctor? Doctors have abdicated their responsibility to cure but they can only work within the boundaries set for them, using the tools and medical education they are provided with. If a Doctor's education is narrow and limited, so will be his practice. It does not matter how brilliant they are *(and many*

Doctors ARE brilliant), **doctors are incentivized, by carrot or stick, to treat and not cure.** To dismiss alternatives, not investigate and embrace them. Doctors excel at managing symptoms but are ignorant of how to heal. Sadly, it is the nature of ignorance the ignorant are unaware they are ignorant!

Remember when they used to give drugs for temporary relief? In the space of a decade whole populations have shifted to taking them for life. Who benefits? The Doctor is happy. He is kept employed and rewarded. Health Corporations are happy, their owners reap stupendous profits. More so when diseases progress to Cancer, heart disease and severe disability. *(Patients pay more when they think they are going to die).*

How about you? Are you happy financing your Doctor's BMW while you struggle to afford a wheelchair? Are you happy taking synthetic chemicals for the rest of your days? Pills which never cure, only prevent you taking the needed steps to heal yourself. Let's not beat about the bush. Until you address its underlying cause, your disease WILL progress.

Doctors tell you to improve your diet, yet know nothing of nutrition. Millions are getting sick and fat, following government **Food Pyramid** guidelines, heavily influenced by the meat and dairy industry. Despite their infatuation with science, Doctors do not know how the body works. If they did, they would not be dying from the same diseases we get. If Doctors knew how to prevent or cure Cancer, they would not get Cancer and if they did, would be able to cure it in themselves. But they do and they can't. So why would anyone with Cancer, seeking a cure, go to a conventional Doctor? With ANY 'incurable' disease, for that matter?

Patients, frustrated with Doctors failure, are increasingly looking elsewhere, turning toward CAM (Complementary or Alternative Methods). Some Doctors, too. The coming together of conventional and alternative systems is known as **Integrative Medicine. Functional Medicine** is another promising development. 40% of patients in the U.S. are enjoying safe, non-toxic, non-invasive treatments that support the body, not burden it. Examples are Acupuncture, Homeopathy, Osteopathy, Chiropractic and Herbalism. These methods can be very helpful. Unfortunately, they aren't being applied correctly *(I explain why, later),* so rarely cure chronic, degenerative disorders.

In Germany, **German Biological Medicine** has grown out of Doctors' greater freedom to innovate. This highly complex system draws on different systems of healing: – ancient, modern and alternative. There is no attachment to a particular modality and practitioners are not forced to stay within rigidly imposed boundaries. This approach makes perfectly good sense. I adopted a simpler version to cure my own disorders.

What about pills? A multi-billion dollar, over-the-counter (OTC) supplements industry has grown up to meet consumer demand for instant fixes, which are not only useless but fraudulent. As a result we end up returning to our Doctors, still sick, poorer in pocket, with a cynical view of alternatives.

Then there is the most important factor in WHY we get sick and how we can recover. We all make excuses but let's face it. The reason we are sick is due to the choices WE make, each and every day.

Each time we choose to consume junk food, sweet biscuits or sweetened sodas, we create imbalance, a nutritional deficit and disease within our bodies. Each time we fail to exercise, we create stagnation and toxic accumulation. Each time we are rude, negative, angry or fearful, deceitful, lacking in love, compassion and consideration for ourselves and our fellow man, we are creating conditions for psychological and physical disease to take hold and, dare I suggest, in this godless age, spiritual death.

Given a choice between fresh fruit and a sticky bun, we turn our noses up at the fruit and opt for the bun. The fruit is building health *("an apple a day…")* while the bun is building disease. We choose disease, even when we **know** the fruit builds health. For any biological species this is insanity. We are committing suicide with our forks and do not seem to know or care. Not only are we killing ourselves but also our children. Guaranteeing, in them, the same chronic diseases we are suffering. Remember when they called it adult-onset diabetes? No more. Now babies are being **born** with diabetes. Sadly, too many parents are psychologically divorced from actions that harm their children.

What about Mental Health? The numbers are staggering. 25% of Americans have some kind of mental disorder. 1 in 4 of the population. There is reason to doubt many of these diagnoses but how many are due to a deficiency of Zoloft, Prozac, Xanax or Ativan? None. 6 million children in America *(and increasingly in the UK)*, who should be outside, climbing trees, are forced to sit in grey, concrete, confinement centres, known as schools, to be drilled and indoctrinated. When they show signs of boredom and restlessness, they are given Ritalin (methylphenidate), classified by the **Drug Enforcement Administration** as a Schedule II narcotic. The same classification as cocaine, morphine and amphetamines. So much for the 'War on Drugs'.

Most of these children are raised in poverty, their bodies and minds poisoned by vaccines, chemical sugars and subversive messages to 'do what you want'. Have you watched children's cartoons? How characters like 'Spongebob Squarepants' plant bad behaviour and 'attitude' in the minds of the young. Messages to defy parents. To demand what is bad for them. Every cartoon filled with burgers, hot dogs, sodas and ice-cream. The brainwashing is not even subtle. It's the same with infant educational material.

The effect on developing minds and nervous systems, from this toxic assault, is devastating. An assault which has been going on for decades. Sick, addicted parents are spawning sick, addicted children. Decent, caring parents are cynically undermined by a corporate mass media, instilling 'needs' in the young, for profit, their health be damned. Humanity is being flushed down the evolutionary toilet. We are the most diseased generation in the history of mankind. The scale of disease is such it can be no accident. In every aspect of our lives there is a pernicious agenda at work. Garbage in, garbage out. The solutions we are presented with do not work and, on closer examination, are crafted to do even more damage.

Do you really think President Obama's much-vaunted '**Personalized Medicine**' initiative is going to cure anyone? Genetics is only one facet of who we are. Perhaps 1% in significance. Genetics gives us the blueprint for building a body but who is the project manager? Who gives it life? Who or what decides whether a gene is turned on or off? What does genetics have to do with someone who cannot afford to eat healthy food and has no choice but to purchase nuggets, sodas and fries? What does the science of genetics have to do with how we think or what we believe? The decision whether to exercise or flop on the sofa, to be violent or peaceful? Half of America has diabetes, 75% are obese, and we focus on genes, instead of locking up the corporate owners who have brought this about.

What kind of sick civilization allows the poisoning of hundreds of millions so a handful of parasitic 'Masters of the Universe' can enjoy obscene wealth and lord it over us? Why isn't the money spent on genetics, conquest and bailing out corrupt bankers, being used to ensure uncontaminated soil, healthy food and decent housing? How much would it cost to take the millions of acres set aside for cattle and plant superfoods? Genetics is going to make already wealthy owners even richer and you can be sure who will be paying the price. You and I. Criminal, corporate America is showing the rest of the world what lies in store for them. I dread to think about the health of future generations.

Do not misunderstand. There are cures out there. I am going to tell you about them. There are healers out there. I have encountered them. Compassionate men and women who have taken patients, sent home by hospitals to die, and cured them, with safe, natural methods. The word 'incurable' not in their vocabulary. Dr Max Gerson and his inspirational daughter, Charlotte, have been healing Cancer, heart disease and other serious conditions, since the 1930s. Dr Gerson cured **Nobel Prize winner Albert Schweitzer** of Type II Diabetes, and his wife of tuberculosis, at a time when TB was taking thousands of lives and considered incurable. Schweitzer said of Max Gerson...

"...I see in him one of the most eminent geniuses in the history of medicine."

Praise indeed. Yet why had I never heard of him and why was I not taught about him in school and why are Doctors not offering the same cure Albert Schweitzer received? When you read Max Gerson's Wikipedia page, as people researching will, it is so damning you want to lock him up and throw away the key. The message is clear. The man is a 'charlatan', his methods 'quackery' and just in case you were thinking of giving his 'unproven' ideas a go, doing so might kill you. One might wonder, if Dr Gerson was curing tuberculosis and cancers when other Doctors couldn't, who exactly the 'quacks' are?

'Hit-pieces' such as this are standard fare on mainstream sites, who condemn the speck in an Alternative's eye, while ignoring the plank in its own. When you have seen enough of them, it becomes easy to recognize the tactics used to keep us away from competition. Sadly, too many, including Doctors, believe what they read.

20 years ago I won a nationwide Information Technology award. Next to the birth of my children it was my proudest moment. Head-hunters called, offering lucrative positions. My financial future was secure. I turned them down. Partly out of loyalty to my employer but mostly because I was 'burnt-out'. Taking anti-depressants just to be able to sleep.

This is something I rarely see talked about. The effects of chronic illness on families. On relationships and budgets. On carers and careers. I have just come off the phone to a young lady whose father is in intensive care with severe health problems and no insurance. The family have expended their life savings on medical bills and are going deep into debt to save him. With each intensive care intervention, the debts mount. This, when the daughter has just undergone a double mastectomy for breast cancer. My heart goes out to her and her family. The effects of sudden and serious illness can be catastrophic.

I wish my mother had known about Dr Max Gerson. I wish my father, who died at 54, from diabetes-related heart failure, had known about Dr Dean Ornish. I wish I had known of Linus Pauling and Dr Abram Hoffer who, 50 years ago, were using nutrition to cure psychiatric and physical disorders. I wish I had discovered earlier, the fascinating, traditional Ayurvedic healer who, in a small clinic, in an Indian backwater, cured my arthritis. Most of all, I wish OUR doctors knew how to cure. It would have saved me years of physical and mental torment, the breakup of my family and the end of my career.

Someone I do know about is Dr Richard Schulze, Naturopath and Master Herbalist. Richard secretly healed patients, for twenty years, before he was forced to stop practicing. He believes absolutely... "THERE ARE NO INCURABLE DISEASES". This colossus of natural healing would see patients four months after they were given only two months to live... the worst of the worst... and cure them. His '**Save Your Life**' video series is a veritable treasure chest of natural healing techniques. Not everyone cares for Richard's outspoken honesty and 'radical' methods but there is no doubting his ability to heal, his vast experience and his power to motivate. He would be the first person I would ask for, if seriously ill.

A less controversial colossus is Linus Pauling, winner of two Nobel's and one of the founders of **Orthomolecular Medicine**. Wiki says of Dr Pauling...

'...one of the most influential chemists in history and ranks among the most important scientists of the 20th century.'

Praise indeed. Linus Pauling surely knows what he is talking about. So I bring up the Wiki page on Orthomolecular Medicine. What does it say?

'...a form of food faddism and even quackery.'

'...untested'

Rounding off the mugging,

'...some vitamins have been linked to increased risk of cancer and death.'

Goodness. Who would try high dose vitamin therapy after reading that? But hold on a moment. Read that last sentence carefully. It is clever and misleading. What does 'linked' mean, exactly, and who linked it? Did they use natural, whole vitamins? Most high street vitamins are synthetic, inorganic fractions of vitamins. Notice they don't say exactly **which** vitamins, so you will likely avoid them all. 'Increased risk' is not quantified. Is that minor risk or major?

Let's try a little linking, ourselves. Imagine someone is killed in a collision with a truck. The driver had fallen asleep at the wheel. It might be reported like this…

'A truck driver fell asleep at the wheel, killing an innocent pedestrian'.

Now let's link the accident to something we wish to undermine…

'A truck driver who fell asleep at the wheel, killing an innocent pedestrian', had been taking Vitamin C.'

The implication, clearly, is the accident was somehow related to Vitamin C. How much greater would be the emotional impact if he had killed a bus full of handicapped schoolchildren? What would happen if **every** media outlet questioned the use of Vitamin C and fabricated even more harrowing stories? Perhaps using paid actors, holding placards, in the TV network's car park, tearfully, demanding Vitamin C be banned from sale.

The media constantly manipulate our emotions, like this, to drive home desired messages. You may recall the huge media fuss about 'stranded' Polar Bears, **linked** to global warming. They failed to mention Polar Bears are excellent swimmers and were doing rather well at the time. Polar Bear numbers were increasing.

Let's try again, this time turning the tables on the corporations. Most store-bought Vitamin C is derived from genetically-modified corn. To cast doubt upon genetic modification, report as follows…

'GM corn linked to truck road death!'

See how easy it is? Now 'link' to any alternative practitioner, practice, or product, you wish to undermine.

In my opinion, Linus Pauling, Max and Charlotte Gerson, Richard Schulze, Dean Ornish and others like them, are heroes, meriting the highest accolades and widest possible exposure, for their contributions to healing. Instead, they remain largely unknown, their methods given little or no official acknowledgment, unless to undermine or misrepresent practitioner or therapy. It is almost impossible to find such healers in western industrialized nations. They operate in secret, or abroad, because they are not allowed to practice at home. They can teach, sell books and supplements. Those who are allowed to practice, may only do so, once modern medicine has abandoned a patient. This is medical dictatorship. There is no health freedom when only a medical doctor can use the words 'cure', 'treat' or 'prescribe'.

When I fired my doctor and travelled to other countries, seeking cures for my own disorders, so impressed was I by the healers I met, and so astounded by the simplicity of their methods, I decided to learn how they did it, so I could help others. Now, because there is such great need in society, it is time to add my voice to those who have gone before and share my knowledge with you. You need to know what you are doing wrong, so you can put it right. You need to learn to be your own doctor because YOU are the one who makes all the choices. Nobody else. If you do not learn how to take care of yourself and your loved ones... knowledge we all used to have... you are lost. We all are. My heart goes out to those who have searched in vain for help. Who have listened to 'expert' opinion and abandoned hope, believing nothing can be done.

DO NOT BELIEVE THEM!

Recovering one's health does not have to be complicated. All you need is a clear understanding of what steps to take and the will and motivation, not only to get started, but to succeed. To end all those years where you have said to yourself, day after day, week after week, month after month,

"Tomorrow. I will definitely start tomorrow".

Do you tell yourself, *"It is too difficult"*? Are you de-motivated by previous failure? Banish these thoughts, look in the mirror and ask yourself a simple question.

"DO I WANT TO LIVE OR DO I WANT TO DIE?"

If you choose life, the knowledge and ideas in this book will help you. If you want to die, please continue on your way and may whichever God you worship, bless your journey. You DO want to live, don't you? That's why you bought this book.

"Do not let either the medical authorities or the politicians mislead you. Find out what the facts are and make your own decisions about how to live a happy lIfe and how to work for a better world."
- Linus Pauling

Chapter 2
Approach with Care

The Internet is the new enlightenment. Unlike my parent's generation, who received information through tightly controlled news outlets, the internet presents us with a great deal more information, good and bad. Enabling us to make more informed choices. It is a marvellous healing tool, relieving symptoms of ignorance in those who use it, wisely. Sadly, it has its downside, revealing things we really wish we didn't know. If you have spent time online, searching for health solutions, you will almost certainly have encountered the unpleasant side of research. A veritable army, paid and unpaid, await the unwary. Their remit? To dissuade the public from trying alternative therapies and keep them in the conventional, corporate-medicine fold. Armed with the 3D's... Disrupt, Defame and Deter... they are a menace to open discussion. You may have encountered them. Natural healing sites; personal or natural health blogs; health-related Facebook groups; internet community forums. They are easy to identify.

Do not be intimidated. There are ways to deal with them. Keep quietly speaking your truth. Never react with anger. Block or use them. Here's how. Every time they react to a post from you, your post goes back to the top of the list. Knowing this, every time they try to attack you, post additional information for others who may be reading. That way, you get the 'bashers' working for you. Or simply ignore them.

Also to be approached with care, are impressive-sounding Consumer Protection websites and 'Scientific' health blogs. They like nothing better than sticking a scientific boot into 'quackery'. Most are industry fronts, using deception and deflection to mislead. What do I mean? An example of deception is when you read an alternative therapy, or product, has not been properly tested. They use terms like:

"No trials". "Unscientific". "Unproven".

The implication is this is bad. Like Pavlovian pups, trained to respond to a negative stimulus, we steer clear and stay within the conventional fold. We have been deceived in three ways.

1. **Omission**. What they don't tell you is natural compounds will never be tested by orthodox medicine because they cannot be patented. Nor can the system test natural methods of healing. There are too many variables (more on this later).

2. **Lies**. Natural healing has been tested over hundreds, if not thousands of years. Personal testimony, case studies, trial and error and simple observation are evidence. Studies also exist. You just do not know where to find them.

3. **Deflection**. Whatever you accuse the other guy of doing is what YOU are doing. We see this all the time in politics. Accuse the targeted nation/leader of wanting to 'take away our freedoms', as you take away theirs. I won't dwell on deceitful politics but you get the idea. In medicine, accuse your competition of not having tested their products, even though your OWN products and methods are largely untested. The **Randomized Control Trial (RCT)** is a relatively recent innovation. 100 years of prior medical practice has yet to be subjected to RCTs. It won't be. It is too expensive to do so and estimates suggest at least 50% of existing medical practice would fail clinical trials. While individual drugs may have been tested, most do not undergo long-term safety tests. Combinations of pharmaceutical drugs, which many of us now take, more so the elderly, have never been tested. Likewise, thousands of synthetic chemicals on the market. In other words:

"No trials". "Unscientific". "Unproven".

Then there is the criminal practice of physicians routinely writing "off-label" prescriptions. Treating conditions with drugs for which there is no evidence or official approval.

"No trials". "Unscientific". "Unproven".

IBM has impressive, futuristic, online medical software, called **Watson Health**. On its website the video introduction informs us:

'50% of medical decisions are not evidence-based.'

'Medical data is expected to double every 75 days until 2020'

It's somewhat ironic medical professionals parrot the meme *"Alternatives lack evidence"*, when their own methods *'lack evidence'*. In 2011, **Scientific American** reported:

'Only a fraction of what physicians do is based on solid evidence from Grade-A randomized, controlled trials; the rest is based instead on weak or no evidence and on subjective judgment. When scientific consensus exists on which clinical practices work effectively, physicians only sporadically follow that evidence correctly.'

A 'fraction'. Yet sites like 'Quackwatch' are nowhere to be seen. If they were to shine a light on the failings of corporate medicine, as much as they do alternatives, there would be a revolution in the morning.

They won't, of course. That's not their purpose. You can't help but sympathize with Doctors, who are as overwhelmed by information as we are.

There is a serious problem with 'Standard Practice'. This is official guidance on the best treatment for a particular disease or disorder. Great if you are really getting the best treatment. Doctors are forced to use treatments they know to be harmful, or useless. On pain of losing their license to practice. Allopathic medicine can take decades to change practices in response to health advances or harmful findings. This means surgeries and treatments, are conducted, that are outdated, of little value, or cause harm. 'Standard Practice' is the Medical Associations' method of forcing conformity and shutting out competition.

Care must be exercised when encountering zealots. These are people who have never tried an alternative therapy, know nothing about them, and yet howl in outrage if you suggest they might have merit. Their attitude is ignorant and irrational. If my car stops working and the garage cannot fix it, I take it somewhere else. People would think me silly NOT to. Yet, if I go to my Doctor and he can't fix my body, or mind, and I go elsewhere, I am committing a cardinal sin. It does not matter if their products are 'not fit for purpose'. It does not matter that my body and health decisions are none of their damn business. I must stick with what doesn't work and not go near those *'dangerous'* alternatives. Even when you point out the shocking numbers killed and injured by modern medicine and contrast it with the total **lack** of harm, from natural or alternative methods, they still fume and fulminate.

What kind of dysfunctional thinking is willing to see human beings die rather than allow them access to safer alternatives which may work? Oncologists **know** chemotherapy does not work on most cancers, injures and kills millions, yet prescribe it anyway. How is this not a criminal act?

I understand why Doctors think like this. 12 years of medical and ongoing education, influenced by drug companies and medical associations, drums into you alternative medicine is *'quackery'* and practitioners are *'kooks'*. Scientific medicine is *'state of the art'*, while old medicine is superstition and blood-letting and medicine-men with bones through their noses. Those cured, without the intervention of a Medical Doctor, are *'spontaneous remissions'* and not healed as a result of their own efforts. Alternatives are *'dangerous'* because they seduce you away from *'proper'* medicine, which will keep you alive, even if it cannot cure you. Faced with this level of indoctrination, you are guaranteed to be met with scepticism and hostility.

An example of Big Pharma's influence over Doctors is the **Merck Manual**, otherwise known as *'The Doctor's Bible'*. It is produced, not by Doctors but a drug company. Rest assured *(cough... cough...)* there is no conflict of interest. Merck is the drug company which produced Vioxx, estimated to have triggered the deaths of 120,000 victims before it was withdrawn. Merck knew Vioxx doubled the risk of heart attacks, yet hid the fact. A deeper investigation of the scandal revealed a variety of criminal and unethical practices by the company, including the intimidation of investigators.

Merck is likely to be involved in a bigger scandal over Gardasil, a vaccine supposedly preventing cervical cancer, which two of its leading Doctors have suggested will eventually become recognized as *"the greatest medical scandal of all time"*. **Dr. Bernard Dalbergue** denounced its approval and continued use, claiming 'everyone' involved with it knows it is completely worthless. Damage inflicted by Gardasil? Sudden death, paralysis, encephalitis, Guillain-Barre syndrome and a host of other ailments. Merck also publishes the **'Veterinarian Bible'**, using the same marketing model to push vaccines and drugs on pets.

I mustn't leave out patients. If you have been taking Statins for 15 years, all the while believing they are protecting you, and someone points out you have been misled, you will come out, all guns blazing, to 'shoot the messenger.' Older guests and callers are like this. They were raised to be trusting of the State and cannot believe the health industry would knowingly cause harm. They come around, eventually, since its failings are increasingly being exposed.

Whatever happened to 'evidence-based' medicine? One of the obvious studies to conduct is to compare disease rates between vaccinated and unvaccinated. Yet, when Congressman Bill Posey questioned the CDC, at an **Autism Congressional hearing** in November 2012, the CDC admitted they had **never conducted a study in the U.S. comparing vaccinated with unvaccinated children**. Studies, using questionnaires, HAVE been conducted in New Zealand and Germany, showing a **5x greater occurrence of common disorders** in vaccinated children, than unvaccinated.

"There are two ways to be fooled. One is to believe what isn't true; the other is to refuse to believe what is true."
- Soren Kierkergard

Chapter 3
Open Your Mind

I cannot know what you already know but if you have made it this far, WELL DONE. You are demonstrating you are serious about resolving your health issues and transforming your life. I understand when you purchase a book such as this you are seeking a cure and want to get right to the bit that tells you how to achieve it. It should be EASY, work QUICKLY and be AFFORDABLE. If you could just pop a pill, or herb, without doing anything else, fantastic! Or ask me to send you the contact details of the Naturopath who confidently stated he could have cured me in 3 days. *(I promise I will share his cure with you, later)*.

Our desire for a 'quick fix' is understandable. We have been conditioned, from childhood, to expect it. Reality is less accommodating. While there are miraculous cures… and you will read of some in these pages… you have tried the 'magic bullet' approach and it has not worked. You may have tried the herb approach and found that has not worked, either. You need to understand, more often than not, you are on the right track but failed to grasp WHY these methods have not worked. The good news is, once you understand what you are doing wrong, herbs and acupuncture, etc., WILL work.

Let me start with what is NOT in the book. I promised friends I would avoid too much technical detail and medical jargon and keep it simple. There are a few sources listed at the back of the book. Those, seeking more detail, know where to look.

There is a wealth of information in the book. If I include every sub-heading in the **Table of Contents** the list would be impractical. There are 46, just for Chapter 29: CURES.

In the book I explain what is making us sick so we can begin to reverse it. Why Doctors cannot cure, so you know it is a dead-end. I recount my own health struggle since you will learn much from it. Then explain, in a way that is easy to understand, why the program I used to heal myself has a better chance of success than anything else you may have tried.

When people are faced with information, challenging their beliefs, 96% will resist, even to the point of violence. I mention this because some of you will not agree with everything I write. Particularly, if your experience of modern medicine has been positive. I do not apologize. The scale of sickness in the U.S. and around the world is a planetary emergency. Unless you are shocked into awareness you will NOT pay attention, stick to a healing program or alter your disease-inducing ways.

Fear works. Ask the Cancer Industry, who do not shy away from using fear to drive patients through their doors. Ask the media. Insiders call regular media fear campaigns, like H1N1, SARS and Ebola, 'cattle drives'. The latest is the Zika virus, blamed for birth defects, instead of hazardous chemicals being sprayed over local water sources, in Brazil.

I long ago turned off the TV, tuning the political and media fear-mongering cowboys out. I had no choice, really, as the extent of 'fake news' coming from government, military and corporations, is simply ludicrous. My world is a far happier place as a result. Listening to those sewing conflict, spreading disinformation, telling me... day in and day out... who I am supposed to hate; which peoples our sons in the military are expected to murder; which twerking, satanic pop diva *(wearing a crucifix while grabbing her thrusting crotch)* our pre-teen daughters are supposed to emulate; and which 'dark', blood-drenched, Hollywood 'blockbuster' I am supposed to applaud, is hardly uplifting. Having said that, fear only motivates for a short period. When, what we are taught to fear fails to materialize, people stop caring. Until the next media hobgoblin is released to frighten us.

We do not use fear to motivate. We eliminate it. **Progress** becomes your motivation. When you start to feel alive again, when your depression lifts, when you throw open the curtains in the morning and shout to the world...

"I FEEEEEL Great!!!"

There is no room for fear. It has been replaced with hope and renewal and gratitude. In my experience of leading yoga, detox and healing retreats, over many years, it takes only 4-5 days to start feeling vital and alive, even after decades of feeling awful.

My intention, in writing this book, is to open minds. Presenting you with accurate, up-to-date information from the health industry's own published data. I do not claim my approach to health is the only way. Or even my way. I give credit where due and pay homage to the great healers of yesterday and today, whose teachings have stood the test of time and from whom I draw inspiration. Their guidance is badly needed in this horribly corrupt age. If you disagree with anything I present, let me know. If I agree with you, I will wear sackcloth and ashes for a week and make corrections. Until then, take what is useful and discard what is not.

Areas addressed in the book

- Why your Doctor will NEVER cure you
- Why Alternatives COULD cure but don't
- The journey from sickness to health
- What you can do to cure yourself

You will find a host of useful insights to help you make better health choices. No need to do as I did, travel the world seeking cures, spending thousands of dollars and countless hours on research. Wading through complex documents, becoming confused and frustrated. Feeling helpless, when faced with contradictory views, from a bewildering number of self-proclaimed experts. Inside, you will find:

- Forgotten and suppressed healing knowledge
- A simplified view of health
- The one step missing that is the KEY to success
- A safe, practical program for healing you can do at home

By the time you reach the last page, something inside you will have changed. You will have new hope; will no longer be confused or dependent on others. You will be your own Doctor. By the way. When you choose health over disease, prepare for attention. People will see the change in you and want to know how you did it!

'The whole aim of practical politics is to keep the populace alarmed (and hence clamorous to be led to safety) by menacing it with an endless series of hobgoblins, all of them imaginary.'
- H.L. Mencken

Chapter 4
"Why Am I Sick, Doc?"

"Why am I sick, Doc?"
"It's Genetic", says the Conventional Doctor.
"Leaky Gut", says the Alternative practitioner.
What a great way to answer the question. Instead of being honest and saying, "I haven't a clue", practitioners make something up. You can understand why. We demand to know what is wrong and expect Doctors to have the answer.

It used to be believed our genes determined whether we would fall ill or not. There was pretty much nothing we could do about it. We could lead a healthy life and still get sick. Our genetic blueprint could not be changed. Now we know genes can be switched on and off. This is called gene expression, the science of 'Epigenetics'. What switches them on or off? Lifestyle. The choices we make every day.

Dr James Chestnut, a popular speaker on health matters, provides a neat analogy of how suspect the *"It's genetic"* answer is. How many times have we seen rivers, lakes and oceans, heavily polluted by oil or chemical spills, with millions of dead and dying birds, fish and seals washed up on the shoreline? Imagine the health sector springing into action. Pharmaceutical drugs would be tossed into the water and mini hospitals set up on the shores of lakes, using tiny tools to cut out tumours and body parts, before the birds and fish die. Eminent doctors, faced with poisoned wildlife, gravely announce, *"It's genetic."*

Now apply this scenario to us. 100lbs overweight, with high blood pressure, high blood sugar, high cholesterol, cancer, heart disease, diabetes, digestive disorders and lung problems. Caused by toxic food, toxic relationships, a lack of exercise and a poisoned environment. Your Doctor tells you, *"It's genetic."*

In what way is this credible?

It is a mutually satisfying game to play. The Doctor maintains an aura of competence. The patient goes home, does not have to make any lifestyle changes, tells everyone they are not responsible for their disease and can do nothing about it, while happily tucking into a box of donuts. Why would Doctors bother with cures, or you change your disease-inducing ways, if you believe the same?

Symptoms of 'Leaky Gut' are so varied you can understand why alternative practitioners diagnose it. The diagnosis has some merit.

Hippocrates said, *"All disease begins in the gut"*. Many are suffering digestive disorders due to the Frankenfood we are consuming.

Research suggests the average medical doctor gets upward of 20% of diagnoses wrong. 30% of those result in death or serious injury. Alternative practitioners are worse. Hardly surprising when symptoms are so vague. Instead of saying they do not know, practitioners diagnose a disorder which has lots of symptoms. If you wish to recover from disease, do not accept this. You are sick because the choices you make have upset the natural balance within your body. You are sick because you have been building disease and not health. You are sick because you have violated Natural Laws. You are sick because you have handed over responsibility for your health, and the health of your children, to people who know nothing about you.

You lack knowledge and have forgotten how to take care of yourself. Parents, whose children have gone through Vaccine Damage Courts, are clearly not responsible for whatever disease passed through a needle, to their children. Although, had they known the true history of vaccines and listened less to pharma-bought officials and media, they may have thought twice about allowing them, looking instead at building natural immunity, which lasts a lifetime.

Regarding general health. In 2013, the **U.S. National Institute of Health (NIH)** reported:

'The United States is among the wealthiest nations in the world, but it is far from the healthiest. For many years, Americans have been dying at younger ages than people in almost all other high-income countries. This health disadvantage prevails even though the U.S. spends far more per person on health care than any other nation'.

For life expectancy, obesity, diabetes, heart disease, COPD (lung disorders), HIV and AIDS, drug deaths and sexually transmitted diseases, America ranked, or came close to ranking, the sickest country out of 17 high-income nations. A staggering 60 million adult Americans, diagnosed with a mental disorder. The United Kingdom is not far behind. Poor health was no longer occurring towards the end of people's lives, when one might expect it, but throughout their lives.

Top reasons presented why so many Americans were sick:
- Too many calories
- Inadequate Health Care
- Poverty, especially child poverty
- Lack of exercise
- Drug abuse

- Poor education

In truth, there were so many reasons it would have been easier to say 'almost everything'. America's health has been deteriorating at an alarming pace. The prescribing rate for drugs in the U.S. has gone up 55x since the 1960's and keeps increasing. This steep incline shows those suffering chronic conditions are not recovering but staying chronic. The NIH report concluded that, unless action was taken to improve matters, levels of illness in the U.S. would only get worse.

Running quickly through the NIH list:

Too Many Calories

I call these 'Diseases of The Fork'. Either 'diseases of affluence', from eating too much rich food, or 'diseases of poverty', from eating low quality food. Both involve far more than just 'too many calories'. World-wide, 60% of all deaths are diet-related.

Inadequate Health Care

Access to high quality treatment is limited to those who can afford it. Remote areas, and crime-ridden inner cities, struggle to attract quality medical staff. Alternative health solutions are not allowed to compete. A system which does not take prevention seriously and fails to address underlying cause, is clearly inadequate.

Diseases of Poverty

"Social inequity kills at an alarming rate", WHO 2009. Malnourishment, environmental and financial stress; poor hygiene; dangerous or dirty occupations. A lack of access to health care, leading to higher rates of infant and childhood illnesses and higher mortality rates; exposure to household chemicals; hidden or untreated infection.

Lack of Exercise

Physical inactivity is a primary cause of at least 35 chronic diseases. Circulation is reduced, you lack proper oxygenation; acid and other wastes are not excreted efficiently; muscles waste and you are not burning excess calories. As actress Helen Hayes informs us... **"If You Rest, You Rust!"**

Drug Abuse

I regard any substance you are addicted to, or using to self-tranquillize, as a 'drug'. That includes food, alcohol, smoking, gambling, sex, pharmaceutical and street drugs and even addiction to stress itself (adrenaline-junkie).

Poor Education

A lack of general education, including sex education. The less well educated are more likely to be taken in by marketing tricks, pseudo-science, dubious and unnecessary medical procedures and media fear-mongering. If Knowledge=Power, then a lack of knowledge makes the poor power-less.

Unmentioned causes of disease were:

Lack of Breast-Feeding

Numerous studies strongly indicate significantly decreased risks of infection, allergy, asthma, arthritis, diabetes, obesity, cardiovascular disease, and various cancers in both childhood and adulthood, for those who were breast-fed. Protective elements in breast milk are not found in infant formula. ([1])

Natural Childbirth

During natural child-birth, new-borns pass close to the anus, picking up important antibodies that strengthen the immune system.

'Electrosmog'

Biological effects of electro-magnetic and wireless radiation that surround all electrical devices, power lines, home wiring, mobile phones, radio, TV and WiFi. Leading to Cancers, hyperactivity, concentration problems, anxiety, irritability, disorientation, distracted behaviour, sleep disorders and headaches.

Heavy Metal Poisoning

The accumulation of heavy metals, in toxic amounts, in the soft tissues of body and brain, such as Aluminium, Mercury, Fluoride, Arsenic, Lead, Barium, Cadmium, Uranium and others. All linked to serious illness.

Iatrogenesis

Sometimes called '**Death by Doctor**'. Millions have died or suffered serious adverse effects at the hands of the medical profession and very few people know. Botched or unnecessary surgery; drug side effects; incorrect prescribing; misdiagnosis. America fares particularly badly with over-medication. The U.S. has 5% of the global population yet consumes 97% of global pharmaceutical output. At any one time 70% of the population are taking one medication, with 50% taking two or more.

What impact on America's health and life expectancy does this consumption have? A clue can be found in the 1974 '**Helsinki Business Study**'. Research, over 15 years, compared two groups, with similar heart problems. The first group saw a Doctor once per year, with no medicines and weren't expected to follow advice. The second group were placed on a regimen of beta-blockers, antihypertensive and cholesterol meds. Standard treatment for cardiovascular disease. Unexpectedly, the numbers who died were 4x higher in the treated group, than the non-treated. This completely shattered conventional wisdom. This same treatment is still widely prescribed. The authorities ignored the findings.

Depression is a major cause of illness. 30% of the population will suffer severe anxiety and depression at some stage in their lives. It starts young, often due to family and social stress. Many have more than one disorder. Modern life is all about 24/7 living and stress (keeping up, getting ahead, material wealth) with less and less time to relax. 1/3rd of the population who suffer stress and stress-related diseases are unaware of its causes. Psychiatric drugs injure millions, trigger suicides, while inducing disorders, such as diabetes.

Causes of sickness in society are easy to see and relatively easy to solve. Each of the mentioned causes can be reversed. Improve food, environment and wealth disparity and end the overuse of toxic chemicals, including those used in medicines. Support the family. Provide quality education instead of 'dumbing down' our children *(What on earth is the Kardashians?!)* If the will were there, governments would address these problems, at source, instead of monetizing and criminalizing individual behaviour. 'Carbon Cops' arresting the public for using a toaster, while Corporations swap pollution for a forest in Botswana, and STILL keep polluting, is not only barmy but unjust.

At the individual level, solving health problems becomes a little more complex. Yes, we can exercise more, grow our own fruit and veg, recycle, be kinder to each other and ourselves, form cooperatives and shop at farmers markets. In the 'Bypass Age' people are increasingly doing these things. However, urban dwellers do not have this possibility and most cannot afford it. There will be little change to the nation's health until food and water, provided to cities, improves.

Unsurprisingly, corporate and military contamination of air, food and water, was missing from the report.

How Bad is It?

We are sick and getting sicker. Today, 133 million Americans – 45% of the population – have at least one chronic disease. 54% of U.S. children. 21% are developmentally disabled. The current rate of Autism in boys is as little as 1 in 28.

Chronic disease is the leading cause of death and disability in the United States.

Latest available figures for the U.S. for common disorders

Allergies	50 million adults suffer nasal allergies. Worldwide, allergies among school children are 40%-50%.
Arthritis	52.5 million (22.7%) of adults.
Asthma	18.9 million (8.2%) adults and 7 million (9.5%) children
Alzheimer's	231,900 nursing home residents
Cancer	230,000 women will get breast cancer this year. The same number of men will get prostate cancer. 2 million new cancer cases each year. 1 in 2 men and 1 in 3 women will develop cancer
Diabetes	30 million. 1.9 million new cases each year. 86 million have pre-diabetes
Epilepsy	2.8 million cases
Heart Disease	26.5 million. 1 in 6 men and 1 in 10 women will die
COPD	24 million have impaired lung function
Obesity	70% of adults are overweight or obese
Sinusitis	Affects 13% of adults over 18

Suppressing Symptoms CAUSES Disease

The concept of suppression is well understood in Psychology. We are encouraged to explore our deepest hurts and fears in order to release them. Not 'bottle up' our feelings. Haven't we all encountered someone who keeps it all inside until they explode with rage or violence?

Suppression is also understood in cancer, where emotional healing is an important part of cancer recovery. We have 13 natural urges.

Sleep, cry, sneeze, breathe, belch, yawn, vomit, eat, drink, urinate, ejaculate, defecate and flatulate.

If you suppress any of these urges there are consequences. E.g. suppressing the urge to sleep can lead to insomnia.

Why, then, does modern medicine suppress the body's natural efforts to throw off disease? If you are in pain, the body is telling you something is wrong. If you suppress that pain, there is STILL something wrong, only the pain is no longer there, nagging you to do something about it.

The body creates a fever to kill off invading pathogens and even cancer cells. It creates diarrhoea to clean out your 'pipework', flush out worms or parasites and combat self-poisoning *('auto-intoxication')* caused by constipation or dehydration. It creates a head cold to carry mucus and sinus blockage out of the body. A sneeze, or cough, to eject an irritant. These are signs of health not sickness. What does your Doctor do? Disable these attempts to heal. The pathogen the fever would have burned up is now free to penetrate the deeper tissues and organs, triggering chronic disease. Yes, you obtained relief but the Doctor only kicked the disease can down the road.

Surgeons act similarly. A century ago, medical wisdom decreed certain body parts were superfluous to requirements and surgeons started to cut them out. Appendix, tonsils, gall bladder, spleen, adenoids, foreskins. When your tonsils become inflamed, they don't bother with underlying cause. They simply take a knife to them. Such is our trust and admiration, at their skill, we say, *"Thank you"*. Why? What if there is something in our diet we are sensitive to and our tonsils are warning us, *"Don't eat this"*? Gluten, or peanuts, or baby formula, or dairy, or tobacco? Aren't the tonsils acting as lymph nodes for the upper brain, filtering pathogens? Now the sentry at your gate has been surgically removed, there will be no more warnings. When your appendix is inflamed, perhaps due to food poisoning, the surgeon makes little attempt to save it. Wouldn't injecting antibiotics directly into the local area resolve the infection and save the appendix? Why surgically remove it? Your appendix is part of your immune system, making white blood cells and antibodies. It produces certain chemicals that help direct white blood cells to the parts of the body where they are needed the most. Now it has gone, your immune system is weaker for it. Perhaps our response should be less, *"Thank You"* and more *"Get the heck away from me with that knife!"*

Fevers are not dangerous, if you keep a patient hydrated, or until they reach 107F. Cancers in Germany are being treated using **Whole Body Hyperthermia**, which raises the body's temperature to fever levels. Prostate cancers are being cured using localized high temperatures. Artificial fevers and hydrotherapy were being successfully utilized by Priessnitz in the 1820's. Creating artificial fevers is an important weapon in the natural healing armoury. The '**Cold Sheet Treatment**', part of the '**30 Days to Health**' program, you read about later, does the same.

Nature does not produce fevers, colds, inflamed tonsils, diarrhoea and pain to inconvenience you when are trying to get to work. These are natural and necessary healing reactions. We should let them run their course instead of suppressing them.

Suppression does not cure disease. It CAUSES it.

Chapter 5
The Diagnostic Dance

The average length of time a Doctor spends with you, during an appointment, is 3 minutes. Within 30 seconds he has already made up his mind what is wrong and stopped listening to you. That is a remarkable diagnostic feat. If he or she cannot figure out what is wrong, specialists using MRIs, blood tests, x-rays, CT scans, allergy testing, angiograms, colonoscopy, ultrasound and more, can. My local hospital offers 88 different diagnostic tests. Invasive, harmful, expensive and often misleading. We undergo these tests even when healthy. An army of 'worried well' attend **Well Man** and **Well Woman** clinics, drumming up new business for public and private hospitals.

Drawn in by my 'need to know', I once coughed up for a comprehensive 'Well Man' screening at my local private hospital. Test results came back normal, except my total cholesterol was a little high, according to their 'catch-all' low threshold. According to my 'you-aren't-catching-me-with-your-baloney' threshold, it was fine. Statins were, of course, recommended (profits from Statins are stupendous), which I declined. I have no faith in the **High Cholesterol = Heart Disease** theory, the catch-as-many-as-you-can threshold, or safety of statins.

Alternative medicine is heading the same way, with Applied Kinesiology, Electro acupuncture (VEGA), Darkfield Microscopy, Hair Mineral Analysis and provocation testing, creating opportunities for treatments and the sale of supplements.

There is a risk, in our efforts to understand WHY we are sick, of being led a merry diagnostic dance. Moving from one specialist to another, using different diagnostic tools, checking minor data points, the results of which are invariably inaccurate. The PSA test, an example. If one test flags a problem, further investigation is needed and off we go for more tests.

Sometimes a practitioner is confident what is wrong, only to have a test contradict him, as I found out. I was diagnosed by a specialist in one of the top hospitals in the country, with Celiac Disease, only for a confirmation test to come back negative. I could see his confusion as he suggested more tests. I had seen a dozen other practitioners before him and was getting tired with the expense and constantly changing diagnoses, so thanked him and walked away. It seemed pointless anyway because I already knew he was not going to cure me. In his world, auto-immune disorders are 'Incurable'. That Doctor visit led me to waste years looking for other causes besides Celiac. Neither of us knew his test was negative because I had not eaten any gluten foods for the few days prior to the test. So, no antibodies showed up. Had he asked what I had eaten, I could have told him.

There is a major problem within western countries of 'over-medicalization'. This has been recognized by the **American Board of Internal Medicine** (ABIM) representing more than 350,000 American doctors. In 2012 the ABIM recommended we get LESS medical care. Their concern? Too many wasteful and unnecessary tests, treatments and procedures. In the UK, 1 in 7 operations are unnecessary. The ABIM's recommendation seems to have fallen upon deaf ears. Many Doctors clearly believe we have too many organs and not enough drugs.

Which sadist invented the mammogram? Squash your breast in a mangle once a year and irradiate it? Only a man could come up with such a device. What is wrong with breast cancer screening? Well, to start with, up to 30% of lumps in the breast will disappear on their own, without intervention. More than 1 million women have been subjected to chemo, radiation and mastectomies, with all the consequences that brings, including death, unnecessarily, after mammograms flagged harmless lumps.

According to this 2012 review by **The Cochrane Collaboration**

'...for every 2000 women invited for screening throughout 10 years, 1 will avoid dying of breast cancer and 10 healthy women, who would not have been diagnosed if there had not been screening, will be treated unnecessarily. Furthermore, more than 200 women will experience important psychological distress including anxiety and uncertainty for years because of false positive findings.'

'Over-medicalization' is not the only problem with mammograms. My conclusion, after reading the latest research (known for years in the alternative community) is mammograms cause more harm than good. You can find more information on the 'CancerActive' website or read the latest Cochrane review. (2)

Testing a few data points, out of thousands of possibilities, is a lucrative business. Such tests are set to increase under the proposed **'Precision Medicine Initiative'**, which seeks to identify genes which are markers for disease. You identify a gene, which suggests an increased risk of this or that disorder. If it is decided you are at risk, drug 'therapy' will almost certainly be prescribed to 'protect' you, while you change your heart-unhealthy or cancer-inducing lifestyle. Since no testing is perfect, there are going to be false positives and negatives.

We know genes can be switched off and on, so this huge backing of genetics seems like another corporate money-grab, while giving the patient little health benefit and a whole heap of worry.

"Your genetic test results have come back, Mrs Smith. You have a 65% chance of developing Multiple Sclerosis".

I wonder if Mrs Smith is going to have peace of mind after hearing that. What is clear from this initiative is that public health measures, targeting the obvious causes of ill health – synthetic 'food', pollution, stress, lack of exercise, poor parenting, poverty, and excess sugar, will be ignored in favour of 'Individualized Medicine'. Corporations profit from the genetic test, follow-up tests, treatments and an expanded market for every possible disease. No symptoms now but your genes predict trouble ahead. Mrs Smith, of course, even if the test is accurate, is not going to change her ways. If you cannot change people's behaviour now, what makes you think you can in the future? I confidently predict there will be no improvement in the nation's health and pharmaceutical stocks are a BUY.

Alternative tests do not escape criticism. They also have a high number of false positives. Many, like muscle-response, or VEGA testing, are dependent on the skill of the operator. If a practitioner gives too much weight to the tests, without confirming via symptoms, you may end up with the wrong treatment for the wrong disorder. In these circumstances, testing is damaging, costing time, energy, money and sometimes our lives.

There is another way to approach our 'Need to Know'. Forget it. Diseases can be resolved **without** a diagnosis. In India, Thailand and Hong Kong, the Ayurvedic, Traditional Chinese Medicine (TCM), Homeopathic and 'Nature Cure' Doctors I encountered, could not afford, nor needed, expensive gadgets and tests. They simply got on with the job of **creating** health, knowing, if you apply the fundamental natural healing steps, illness will resolve:

- Clean the body

- Flood it with nutrients

- Exercise

- Reduce stress

The ancients believed a clean body, provided with proper nutrition, would stay healthy. While a dirty body, lacking nutrients, would sicken and die. There were no such things as clinical trials. They observed nature. We do the same inside our homes. Place a houseplant in good soil, give it clean water and watch it thrive and blossom. Transplant it into poor soil and watch it weaken, fail to bloom, and pests and fungi will attack it. Reverse the process and the plant thrives again. The greatest influence on the health of the plant is the quality of its soil. The 'Biological Terrain'.

Where I live, in Thailand, animal welfare activists commendably brought an end to dog meat appearing on the nation's menu. Unfortunately, their success had a downside. The number of stray dogs in the country has exploded. Dogs are everywhere, emaciated and weak, infested with parasites, their skin scaly, fur dry and patchy, often dying from road accidents, neglect and starvation. If you take them in, deal with the parasites and feed them, their bodies fill out and their fur grows back. Add some tender loving care and they thrive. No chemistry. No pathology. No clinical trials. No Ketogenic or fad diet. Just biology and common sense.

Biological laws are the same for us as for houseplants and stray dogs. When our defences are weak, our 'biological terrain' poor, we open ourselves to viral, bacterial, fungal and parasitic infection. We can conduct tests to identify which bacteria, which virus, which microbes, and deal with them but does it really matter we know? Simply clean the body, which includes blood-cleansing and parasite removal, give it the nutrients needed to strengthen defences, and we get better. This natural mode of healing has operated for thousands of years.

I have witnessed, many times, people recover from illness without knowing precisely what was wrong or what cured them. Natural healing is not the same as symptom-based medicine. If you improve your diet, exercise, dissolve emotional stress, take herbs & vitamins, add hydrotherapy, relaxation training, meditation, breathing exercise, acupuncture, a chiropractor and any number of other techniques and your health recovers, how do you know what cured you? It is impossible. Herbal combinations can include multiple herbs, with many different actions, acting synergistically. According to **Dr Duke's Phytochemical and Ethnobotanical Database (3)** Mangosteen, a delicious Asian fruit, has 245 distinct actions on the body. How do you know which actions, or phytochemicals, within Mangosteen, trigger healing? You don't. That is just one fruit. Introduce other supplements and therapies and you have an infinite number of variables. This is the main reason, when researching alternative methods of healing, sceptics describe them as:

"untested", "unproven", "no clinical trials", "not supported by the science"

What they don't tell you, or fail to realize, is it is **impossible** to prove natural healing works, using current testing paradigms. You are not testing one chemical against one symptom.

"Drugs make a well person sick. How can drugs make a sick person well?"
- Abram Hoffer, MD

Christa

72-year old Christa, from Switzerland, was suffering from Type II diabetes and too many years of smoking. You could hear her wheezing when she breathed. After two incidents of collapsing, she learned she had diabetes. Her A1C reading was 7.8 and fasting blood sugar 177. The normal range is 80-100. Above 120 and the body starts to suffer damage. Christa was initially placed on insulin, then Metformin, by her Doctor.

Christa's family were concerned about her health and encouraged her to sign up for our 21-day '**Reverse Diabetes**' program. It is usual to have doubts but these were dispelled when her blood sugar readings quickly reverted to normal. Christa was delighted. A big concern was whether Christa she could kick her smoking habit. This proved to be far easier than she thought, thanks to an herbal tincture that eliminated her cravings. Stopping was a breeze.

Christa came off all her medications. After 20 years of coughing and wheezing, she now breathes easily. Her fasting blood sugars are within normal ranges. She also shed some weight. The retreat was a success, not least because Christa is a remarkable lady. Determined, compliant *(she stuck to her program)*, sociable and easy to look after. Having experienced normal blood sugars and the benefits of fasting, Christa now knows what works.

The Reverse Diabetes program is juice-fasting, with some herbal supplements and light exercise. Followed by a **LCHF** (Low Carb, High Fat), ketogenic diet. Included is the herbal steam sauna and Thai Traditional massage. A treat! Follow-up support helped Christa stay on the straight and narrow.

Chapter 6
Rise of the Health Coach

A million health 'experts' are online. Like town-hall barkers, they vie for our attention and money. The result is noise and confusion. We cannot separate truth from lies, spin from substance. The choices available to us are endless and bewildering. Everything seems to cause everything. Have you noticed? If your disease is not caused by a lack of Vitamin C or D, it is Candida or B12. Echinacea and DX-64 'Bio'-thingamabob can fix it. Purchase Echinacea for $24.99 and all will be well. Until you discover there is NO Echinacea in 90% of over-the-counter (OTC) Echinacea products or the herbs you just purchased are so weak you need 20 capsules a day to feel any effect. With practices like this, how can any of us get well? The poor quality of OTC products is one reason I learned to make my own herbal remedies. Later, I share the secret.

In the last few years, conventional medicine has acknowledged there is a problem with patients not being able to follow instructions given by their Doctors. 50% of patients, on leaving a Doctor appointment, have no idea what their Doctor just told them. If you are being treated with **'German Biological Medicine'**, you can pretty much make that 100%.

The stock advice to change diet, exercise more and reduce stress is not being complied with. How can people be expected to change their unhealthy ways if they do not understand what they are supposed to do and lack support? They need guidance and encouragement, which Doctors do not provide. Doctors believe 99% of patients who need to change their lifestyle, will fail. Clearly we have a problem. Lucky for us, there is a solution. In March 2013 **UK Health Minister** Anna Soubry urged the National Health Service in England, and local teams, to take *"urgent action"* to support Cancer Recovery patients and provide them with a proper Cancer Recovery Plan.

The need for support, not only with cancer recovery, has given rise to the relatively new profession of 'Health Coaching'. In the U.S., Health, Wellness, Life and Fitness Coaches are already part of the landscape. A Health Coach bridges the gap between Doctor and patient. It is an excellent idea. In the UK, **National Health Service (NHS)** nurses are being trained for this role. However, it does not bode well. When Cancer wards and hospital food consists of soda and sugary biscuits, and nurses are being taught there is no difference between organic and processed food, no amount of 'coaching' will restore health. 50% of NHS nurses are obese. These are the people teaching you and I about nutrition!

Health Coaches come in various flavours and with differing levels of expertise and experience. I have adopted the label, championing natural methods, helping those suffering chronic diseases, like cancer, diabetes and arthritis, to reverse or better manage their conditions.

An ideal Health Coach has a broad understanding of healing, knows what works and what doesn't, what supplements are useful and which are not. They understand what you should be eating, what will keep you well and provide encouragement as you make lifestyle changes. Health Coaches work with you, moving you toward health and away from disease.

When people come to me, confused and frustrated, I feel compelled to help. If you have useful knowledge, how can you not? It was never my intention to travel this path. Friends would mention their health problems and were surprised at my knowledge and delighted when I pointed them toward solutions. They had never heard of Ayurveda or Nature Cure, Ornish or Esselstyn, the Thomsonian School of Healing or Father Kneipp, Benedict Lust or Orthomolecular Medicine. They thought a detox was a packet of tea bags and a Princess Diana colonic.

I taught them Yoga but not like they had been taught before. Advanced breathing exercises they never knew existed. Gave weight loss and nutritional advice, tapped on meridians, helped them quit smoking and sobbed with them as emotional traumas were dissolved. Then they started to ask me to design detox and healing programs. To support them as they went through them. To be 'on call' if anything went wrong. To be their alternative medicine and natural healing 'Guru'. I never imagined I would find myself writing health books, leading retreats and providing online guidance. I prefer a quiet life.

There is another reason I never imagined reaching this point. I should be dead. If I had stayed with conventional medical Doctors and Psychiatrists I have no doubt I would have committed suicide or be in a wheelchair, crippled with Arthritis, Celiac Disease, Fibromyalgia, chronic depression and debilitating anxiety. Taking painkillers, anti-depressants, beta-blockers, muscle-relaxants, anti-inflammatories and hypoglycaemia meds. Adding $1.5 million dollars to the corporate balance sheet.

Instead I chose a different future and **Fired My Doctor**.

You can do the same. It's a little scary firing your Doctor. It means flying solo into a bewildering world of complexity and competing claims. If you find you are struggling, for whatever reason, seek help. Track down a Naturopath, Health Coach or call some of the other teachers and holistic practitioners out there doing good work. One conversation really could change your life. Try not to be too hard on them, though. After all, we are coming out of a Dark Age of Medicine where, for the last 100+ years, modern medicine has had its 'Bypass Age'. Bypassing what could heal you, in favour of what could be patented, synthesized and monetized. Cures and exciting research, buried in libraries, suspiciously un-indexed, for 50 years or more, is being unearthed, as a wave of practitioners and researchers resurrect the lost Art of Healing.

It is an exciting time but also worrying. The forces of conservatism will not give up passively. They know every trick in the book. After all, they have had a century of practice. You see it with the health supplements Industry. 'Big Pharma' had no need to duke it out with natural supplement companies, who started eating into their market share. It simply bought them up, converted natural ingredients to synthetic and wrapped them in fancy packaging, at inflated prices. You don't buy a single herb, vitamin, or skin cream, anymore. Now it's a 'Cellular', 'Nutraceutical', 'Bio-Nano', 'Skin-Whitening', 'Anti-Aging' System, with an air-brushed picture of an impossibly-thin, female model, with bleached teeth and a nose-job (in Asia these models look like aliens). You can no longer find skin creams. They are 'serums'. When I see the dazzling cosmetics panels in stores, I shake my head and pass by. The health supplements and cosmetics markets are multi-billion dollar, deceptive-marketing obscenities. I know. I worked in the industry and saw the chemicals used. Some of them so harsh, well-known brands would farm production out to other companies because their workers would get sick. I know how little 'natural' product goes into them. That $100 'serum' you just bought? The ingredients cost $1.

How can people like me help those who feel overwhelmed and confused? Can't you just go straight to an Ayurvedic Dr., Naturopath, or Chiropractor? Absolutely. Just understand, alternative practitioners need to make a living, have mortgages to pay and families to take care of. Unlike your GP, they spend more than three minutes with you. They are not subsidized by the State and do not get free trips to Disneyland, for pushing over-priced meds. Expect them to be more expensive than your Doctor.

Some alternative practitioners have taken a lead from conventional Doctors. They know you are not going to change your ways, so do what conventional Doctors do. Instead of pharmaceutical medicines, they prescribe herbal remedies. These will not harm you but, alone, are unlikely to heal you. That means repeat prescriptions. This is not such a bad thing. If you are not going to change your lifestyle, at least bolster your defences. Herbs can be protective. I call them my 'clean-up' crew. For instance, Milk Thistle protects the liver when you are still drinking. Hawthorn Berry, the heart. Fresh, raw garlic, certain cancers. Bitter herbs can manage diabetes. They will not harm you in the same way pharmaceuticals do. Just make sure there is some actual herb in the bottle and not a weak decoction of leftover twigs, sprayed with pesticides, shipped over, irradiated and gassed, from somewhere in the third world.

The quality of herbal supplements is a major issue. In February 2015, the **New York Attorney General's Office** asked major retailers Wal-Mart, Walgreens, Target and GNC, to halt sales of certain herbal supplements. 79% of their herbal supplements were found to have NO herbal DNA. The worst offender was Wal-Mart, with 96% of their supplements having no DNA from plants listed on labels.

Tens of millions today are suffering chronic degenerative disorders. The only chance they have of reversing their disorders is to change their disease-inducing ways. To detoxify all the poisons and pollutants, improve their diet, reduce stress and get their bodies moving. Changing lifestyle is, literally, a life or death decision. It sounds simple when you see it written down but like New Year Resolutions, which last all of 5 minutes, it is not easy to make lasting changes.

Knowledgeable patients understand they cannot get well without support. An army of health tourists regularly descend upon Detox and Yoga Retreats in Thailand, Malaysia, Mexico and elsewhere. They know, if they undertake programs at home, they will fail. There are too many temptations, distractions and resistance from others. They may also lack knowledge. In an holistic retreat setting – five-star spa or a simple hut on the beach – the support, education and attention they receive is high quality and fundamental to kick-starting lifestyle changes. Many times I hear retreat guests say,

"This is the best thing I ever did for myself".

Not everyone can afford to jet off to sunny climes. This is where the Internet is a saviour. Imagine being able to consult face-to-face with a Health or Wellness Coach, over the Internet, using online video software, like 'Skype', from the comfort and privacy of your living room or office? Calls are free. It certainly beats trudging to the Doctor's surgery, waiting in line on a cold winter's day, for 3 minutes of attention, then walking out, mystified by what you were just told, clutching a bag full of side-effects. Online scheduling software allows you access the Coach's online calendar and select the slot you want.

What kinds of questions do people ask a Health Coach?

They can be basic:

"How do I detox from fluoride?"

Pleas for help:

"My husband is being difficult. Can you talk to him?"

Wailing and gnashing of teeth:

"I am tired of this diet. Can I have a glass of wine and a steak, PLEASE!" *(They know the answer but I commend them for trying).*

Panic:

"I started my detox and am feeling awful. Should I stop?"

Serious:

"Help! I'm trying to come off anti-depressants and am overwhelmed by anxiety and suicidal thoughts!"

Then there is the good stuff that makes it all worthwhile:

"It's unbelievable. My depression has lifted!"

"I feel amazing!"

"All my symptoms have gone!"

"Thank you. You saved me a fortune".

"I had no idea it was so easy!"

Finally, from a friend with diabetes:

"I can see!"

No. I don't cure the blind, nor do I raise the dead. He meant he could see **better!**

If this sounds a little like blowing my own trumpet, of course I am. Yet, there is a serious purpose in sharing examples. People are lost, even though they have access to incredible amounts of information and no shortage of experts. EVERYONE with a keyboard is an expert. Have you noticed? Post a question in a Facebook Group and you will get 150 suggestions. What odds you select the one that heals you?

Experts don't agree with each other and keep changing their minds. No sooner have they made one discovery, a few years later, they overturn it with another. No apology or mea culpa. They simply present the new diet or 'revolution', in a flurry of publicity, without missing a beat.

There are so many options available. Take diets. Where do you even start?! There have been thousands of different diets foisted on the public over the last 100 years. Yet, NOT knowing what to eat can be costly.

If my Naturopathic friend is correct, I could have been cured in 3 days. Instead, it took 20 years. In that period my efforts to recover my health, loss of job and expected future earnings, cost me around £600,000. If I include future income from raises, bonuses and promotions, it could easily be £1 million. I was an Information Technology (I.T.) expert.

Your circumstances may be different but if I had encountered someone who understood the different methods of healing… Modern, Complementary, Alternative and Natural… when I first began to struggle, someone who could advise me what to eat and what therapies to consider, I might have been spared my long ordeal. Do I believe there is benefit in paying for a 'Health Coach'? It depends on who it is. There are good and bad in all professions but if I had my time again, I would be on the phone in a heartbeat. Experience is a powerful teacher.

Who might benefit from a Health Coach?

- Those seeking clarity
- Lacking a healing program or struggling to understand one
- Needing guidance, support and inspiration
- 'Grasshoppers' who hop from therapy to therapy
- Those wanting to check they are being given good advice

At Antarana we never know who is going to walk through our doors and with what set of conditions. It is fascinating how unique is an individual's history, character, personality traits, habits, hopes and fears. They need individualized, customized solutions. Not standardized, complex specializations no-one can understand.

One of our biggest health challenges is taking what we learn and applying it. We are not all motivated, or learn, the same way. Some can be sat with a book open in front of them and an instructional video playing, yet not understand. These types need to be taken by the hand and shown. Stress can play a role I learning. Blocking our ability to take in new information, comprehend what we are seeing, or take action.

Others who come unstuck are those with theoretical knowledge but no practical experience. Their knowledge, even if extensive, remains at the level of the intellect. Some of the prominent speakers I see would not be able to handle bowel cleanses or cope with someone who needs emotional healing. They connect easily with a large audience but struggle one-on-one with someone in crisis. The best practitioners are those who have been through the school of hard knocks and are not simply armed with book-knowledge. The best person to counsel a recovering alcoholic is a recovered alcoholic. The best person to cleanse your body is someone who conducts cleanses (detox). The best person to take you through a healing program is someone who has healed themselves. I even see practitioners, lost and frustrated, who contact me, seeking clarity. It is easy to be overwhelmed.

Theoretical knowledge is fine but how do you, step-by-step, conduct a program and see it through to completion? Many questions can arise.

- Would you recognize a 'healing crisis' and how to respond?
- When cleansing, how do you know when a body is clean?
- What if you cannot find uncontaminated food or supplements?
- Should you keep taking medication the Doctor prescribed?
- What if herbal remedies/vitamins/juices aren't working?

When you purchase a house or business, you will often hear the most important three factors are 'Location, Location, Location.' In health, it is 'Education, Education, Education.' Educating retreat guests and online callers takes up much of my time. Whether it is teaching nutrition, explaining natural methods of healing or recommending which (not 'Witch') Doctor to use. People need help navigating it all.

Over the years I wasted thousands of pounds on tests and treatments that failed to properly diagnose my condition or its cause. Few would have been necessary had I been better informed or had someone independent to ask. Today, with years of research and practical experience behind me, I know pretty much what works and what doesn't. Where I do not know, I know where to look, or will turn to colleagues such as **Paul Johnson, MD.**, a retired Paediatrician and Oxford researcher who, even as I type, is using science to prove the value of ancient breathing techniques in balancing the nervous system. His vast experience and no-nonsense, academic mind can sniff out a 'quack' therapy, instantly.

"In the history of humanity there has never been a disease that someone, somehow, somewhere has not eradicated, removed the disease from their body and totally healed. Can what they did work for you? Is there a reason why it should not?"
*- **Sharon Forrest***

Chapter 7
Nobody Cures You

One of the greatest errors in medicine is the belief someone else cures us. I need to make it clear and you need to understand.

No Doctor cures you

No Alternative practitioner cures you

No Natural healer cures you

Nobody stands over you with a magic wand and says, "Abracadabra! You are healed." The great natural healing systems of the world all understand. THE BODY CURES ITSELF. The goal of all practitioners should be to fire up and support the body's own self-healing mechanism, remove all impediments to healing and provide it with the materials it needs to repair. The body then heals. And when it heals, it does not just heal your Cancer, Heart Disease, Diabetes or Arthritis. It heals all of them. As Charlotte Gerson says,

"You cannot heal one disease and keep two others. When one heals, they all heal".

The focus of natural healing is not so much the disease itself *(the name we give is not so important)* but cleaning and strengthening the body. If you are fortunate and have a good practitioner near you, enlist their help. Many people are not so fortunate. They lack the finances for practitioner fees, healthier diets and/or supplements. In the mainstream, some diseases are exorbitantly expensive to treat. Cancer has bankrupted many, who not only have to absorb the cost of conventional treatment but the cost of recovery, which can also be significant. All is not lost. You can still do some things, such as Yoga, which is free and needs little space or equipment. Or simple stretches and exercises. Fasting and Water Cures *(I talk about these later)* cost pennies. The ancients did not drive expensive cars or have the latest iPhone. In some societies there was no such thing as money or 'medicine'. The medical profession did not exist, yet people healed.

No matter one's budget, if you are suffering a chronic, degenerative disorder, or wish to avoid one, you are going to have to take matters into your own hands, accept responsibility for your disease and do something you have not tried before. **Instead of building disease, build health.** Instead of relying on others, rely on yourself. It is amazing what the body can do, given a chance. Miracles can happen if you believe in yourself. The good news is, for most disorders, healing can happen quickly. The great natural healers will tell you they see patients, sick for decades, throw off their disease in a matter of days. I see it myself, when counselling. With **EFT** and '**Breaking The Chains**', traumas and addictions that have been tormenting people for years, dissolve, in minutes. How is this possible? I could try to impress you with some pseudo-scientific explanation of how these techniques work but often it is simply the first time people have attempted to address the problem. They weren't aware they could.

Within these pages I present a healing program that draws on the simplest techniques from both ancient and modern healing practices. A program that can be conducted at a retreat, cabin in the woods, or in your own home. You can even choose the pace at which you wish to recover. If you are frail, take it slowly. It may take 18 months. If stronger, 6 months. If you are prepared to put in the required effort, you may see results in 30 days or less. It would be wrong of me to claim every disorder is healed, every time. No-one can give such a guarantee. We are all different. However, once you read and understand how the method works, you will see it has the potential to do what it says on the tin.

A **key to successful healing** is not whether a method is unique *(there are many roads to Rome)* but how diligently you apply it. If you are someone who believes your disease or disorder is 'incurable' because that's what the Doctor told you, rid yourself of the idea right now. I personally do not believe Mother Nature is so cruel she would deny us the ability to heal. By the way. It is not going to be as before, with a Doctor dispensing a few pills. Healing is going to require your full participation.

- YOU decide to stop doing whatever is making you sick
- YOU decide what you put in your mouth
- YOU decide to move your body or flop on the couch
- YOU decide whether to remain spellbound by TV, computer or smartphone
- YOU decide to feed your mind useful, or useless, thoughts
- YOU decide whether to act on what you read in this book and see it through to completion

Of one thing you can be sure. If you do nothing, you will stay sick. Nobody is going to come along and sprinkle you with pixie-dust.

100 Doctors

Once Upon a Time there was a powerful King who had 100 doctors. The finest in the land. Soon, one of the older Doctors died and a search began for a replacement. Many candidates came to be interviewed. Each candidate had to correctly answer one question from each of the other Doctors. All failed.

One day a candidate arrived who answered all the questions correctly. The King congratulated him and welcomed him as the 100th Doctor. The Doctor said,

"Your Highness. Before I take up the position, I would like to ask the other Doctors a question".

The King, intrigued, agreed. Addressing the group, the Doctor asked,

"What are the two most important things for health, which cost nothing?"

The Doctors answered. None correctly.

"What are they?" asked the King, intensely curious.

"A walk in the morning and an hour in the sunshine".

So pleased was the King with this answer, he fired all the other Doctors and the new Doctor became the most famous physician of his Age.

This ancient story is a reminder of how, in a world of complex remedies and impenetrable jargon, preventing illness and maintaining our health can be quite simple. The two most important things for health have, arguably, not changed.

Sunshine

We have been taught to fear the sun. This is absurd. Heliotherapy (sun-bathing) is an important part of 'Nature Cure' programs. Vitamin D is crucial for protecting us against cancer. Sunshine on our skin produces it. Sunshine is also an anti-depressant. We feel miserable in the darker months in the northern hemisphere, without it. We need MORE sunshine, not less.

There is no need for us to be fearful of the sun just because some industrialist wants to sell toxic sunscreen and a few Aussies have overdone it. Everything in moderation. Go out in the sun when it is not too high in the sky. Spend an hour, twice daily. Ensure you do not burn. Too much sun, like too much of anything, can be bad for you but so can too little.

Exercise

How many of you take a walk in the morning? When I was in the military, exercise would commence at first light. In the Mediterranean, walking is common, particularly after a meal. There is something magical about the cool early morning air. While the rest of the country is sleeping, an early morning walk is invigorating and ensures greater mental sharpness for the rest of the day. Exercise during the day helps you sleep better at night. It also helps with constipation, reduces the risk of breast and colon cancer, burns calories and gets more oxygen into body and brain. Getting our circulation moving improves sexual health, muscles get stronger and so do the bones of osteoporosis patients. Immune function strengthens, 'bad' cholesterol drops, stress reduces and physical tension is released. Walking briskly each day can reduce your risk of heart disease by 40%.

A morning walk is not so easy when you work shifts, live in a city, do not feel safe outside or only have time for a mad dash to work. Here you must do what you can. Exercise later in the day. If you cannot walk, get on your bike. If you cannot do that, learn some simple breathing and stretching exercises.

One fun Qigong exercise I do each morning is called 'Tossing the Ball'. It is perfect for almost everyone, including the overweight and less mobile. It can also be used to dissolve toxic emotions. Instead of 'tossing' a ball, imagine you are tossing away anger, fear, hatred, heartbreak or frustration. This exercise can be conducted slowly, or at an increased pace, becoming a super workout. It does not need any equipment, costs nothing and you don't have to move from one spot. Search for it online or watch for a future video on the Antarana website.

There is a problem with government guidelines on exercise. The same problem we find with taking medicines, or with the food we eat. We aren't all the same! 20% of people, doing the typical exercise we see in gyms, do not see the benefits they expect. These are called 'non-responders'. 15% do exceptionally well and are called 'super-responders'. The type of exercise chosen needs to be tailored to individual need and response.

You have heard of **Personalized Medicine**. Well, genetic testing is bringing us **Personalized Exercise**. Tests claim to be able to identify whether you are a 'non', 'low' or 'super' responder. These tests also suggest an exercise plan *(for a few dollars more)* but many genetic tests only test one single data point and are unreliable. Buyer beware.

My own reluctance to flogging myself in a gym, is to avoid being in the same company as steroid-munching gorillas, preening hedonists and gay pick-up merchants. I have always been more **Mr Bean** than **Arnold Schwarzenegger**.

Whatever the claims of genetic testing, it is my observation that, no matter the body type, a two week Royal Marine training course will leave everyone bursting with energy. The military have taken millions through rigorous training, over hundreds of years, so you would think they would know about responders and non-responders. Yet, when I served, I never heard of this. You could see who was built for marathons and who was built for speed but all undertook the same exercise and all benefited. Military strength, fitness and endurance training is definitely hard core!

The obvious danger of genetic tests reporting you as a 'non-responder', is we are back to that sorry excuse, 'It's genetic'. If you are told you are a 'non-responder' you won't see any value in exercise at all. Don't surrender too readily. There are numerous health benefits to moving the body, not just aerobic fitness, weight loss or muscle gain. You HAVE to get that lymphatic system moving so it can eliminate waste. When you exercise, try to raise a sweat.

Most people I see are over 50, with dodgy knees and carrying too much weight. They need gentle introductory strength-building programs to get tendons and ligaments ready for more vigorous exercise. Otherwise injury rates are high. This is where yoga is my preferred choice. But you MUST not push yourself beyond your capacity. Don't worry about trying to match the hedonists and advanced students bending their lithe bodies into incredible positions. It took them many years to reach that stage. Think about YOUR body. Don't run before you can walk.

Christians and Yoga

Christianity in the U.S. has a large following while, in the UK, it is very much on life support with less than 4% of the population actively practicing. Christians sometimes worry about Eastern disciplines, like Yoga, concerned they are gateways to worshipping 'false gods', or deviations from living a purely Christian life. Are these concerns justified?

Dr Dean Ornish' Heart Program, which reverses heart disease using diet, exercise and stress reduction, was given to him by a Hindu Swami? Knowing this would you reject it? Is a Hindu REALLY worshipping a 'false' god? Or is he worshipping the many faces of ONE god? The same God you worship?

Many years ago, when dipping a toe in the spiritual waters, I asked a priest if Christianity had an exercise program? It seems an odd question but I had begun to practice yoga and was advised to stay away from it, by the priest, *"Yoga is used by Satan to seduce Christians away from their faith."* This sounded overly dramatic and unlikely. If one's Christian faith is so weak one can be seduced by a towel and exercise mat, perhaps the problem isn't so much Yoga but one's own lack of faith.

The '**New Age**' movement has attracted spiritual seekers, leading to experimentation with astrology, astral projection, crystals, Ouija boards, Tarot, mediums and so on. This I concede is a cause for concern. One might wonder what is so wrong with traditional Christianity people are rejecting it in favour of alternatives? It is an unfortunate reality that any mention of 'Christianity' or 'God', to those who come to see me, will cause their eyes to glaze over and they will be out the door faster than a greyhound out of a trap. In their view, organized religion is discredited. Hardly surprising when you are constantly assailed by stories of priestly paedophiles and religions at war. Please don't get me started on televangelists. You don't need to see a trident and horns to know the 'devil' is at work with these money-grubbing 'false prophets'.

Christian web sites warn 'Namaste', means 'I bow to the god within you.' A billion people on this earth greet each other by clasping their hands together and nodding or bowing in respect, including millions of **Christians** in India. What should a western Christian do? Cause offense and run away, so they are not seen to be 'bowing to another god?' Or simply be courteous and return the greeting? After all, if there IS only one God, how could there be another 'god' within them? I like the Asian way of greeting. It is more sanitary than shaking unclean hands, or wincing from the handshake of some hulking brute that can crush stone.

'Om' is a Sanskrit word, associated with Yoga, which alarms Christians. There is nothing to fear. 'Om' is spelled A-U-M. 'Aum', 'Amen'. 'Aum', 'Amen'. You see? They have the same linguistic root.

I have been practicing and teaching therapeutic Yoga, off and on, for 25 years. Inspired by the man most responsible for the resurgence of modern Yoga in the west, Krishnamacharya. He did not deny the West the benefits of yoga because 'Christians only believe in one God'. Had he done so, we may never have learned this wonderful practice. His attitude toward religion and Yoga was only, *"That we acknowledge a power greater than ourselves."* The religious aspect of Hinduism can be off-putting. His son, Desikachar, studied under him for 28 years, with one condition. No God. Trained as an engineer, he did not want the religious trappings.

Christians can relax. Today, Yoga has largely been stripped of religion. Better yet, turn Yoga into **'Christian Yoga'** by injecting your **own** beliefs into your practice. How might this work? When meditating, use 'Amen' as your mantra. When doing the 'Sun Salute', imagine you are saluting God or Jesus. If a pose or breathing exercise results in the resolution of a physical ailment, or emotional wound, give thanks to God. What matters is your INTENTION.

There are many styles of Yoga. I cut my teeth on Sivananada Yoga before putting together my own program, tailored to my body's capacity and specific needs. I sometimes draw on Iyengar Yoga, which has exercises to treat and prevent a wide range of illnesses. The style of Yoga I teach is better described as 'Yoga Therapy'. It is gentle. Too many people get injured attempting postures their bodies are not ready for. Yoga is a wonderful system which, practiced correctly and safely, brings tremendous benefits.

There is another aspect to Yoga and other non-Christian practices, which fall into the category of 'Spiritual journey' or quest. I would describe myself as a lost soul, or Prodigal Son, who, dissatisfied with life, spent years shopping at the Alternative Healing and Spiritual bazaars. Along the way, I encountered many other lost souls, seeking an alternative to the godless, material, selfish, uncaring world the merchant class has created for us. The class that wants to destroy God because he is 'competition'. The class that has no problem with religion, provided you worship Pepsi, Nike, Exxon or Apple.

Yoga led me back to Christianity by helping me understand my own religion better. It led me back to Christianity because I recognized it would take me 40 years of yoga meditation to achieve what Christian Saints could achieve, overnight, through the power of Grace. Later I provide an example of this.

There are some Yoga practices which lead to transcendent states but very few adherents achieve them. I see the western 'pony-tail and flip-flop brigade' (no offence intended) as seekers. Eventually their seeking will draw them back home.

Do not fear them or for them. Work on yourself instead. Christians are instructed to, 'Let your light so shine that you honour your father in heaven'. Instead of worrying about others, work on shining your own light, so it attracts others to you. Like a moth to a flame.

Greg

Greg was a typical ex-seaman. 70 years old when he had his third heart attack. A seemingly hopeless case, Greg was grossly overweight, smoked, took no exercise, ate meat-pies and chips and loved his sugary mug of tea. He was on assorted heart medications, beta-blockers, statins, etc., convinced they gave him protection. After his third heart attack, Greg finally got the message. If he didn't change his ways, a fourth would be his last.

I saw Greg 7 months later and was shocked by the difference in him. He had lost 25kg (50lbs) and looked vital and alive. Gone was the walking dead man I knew. Greg told me all his blood work was normal, he had stopped his medication and the Doctor said he was out of danger as far as his heart was concerned.

All this was incredibly good news. I wanted to know the secret to this amazing turnaround. Greg told me he could not completely change his lifestyle. Cycling seemed less arduous than pounding the streets, so he purchased a bicycle. What started out as ½ a mile per day, eventually turned into 15. The change in him, from exercise alone, was impressive.

I would like to say Greg lived happily ever after. Not so. 12 months on, Greg's heart gave out. What Greg had not revealed to me, or his Doctor, was he was still smoking.

I mention this story because it is instructive. People commence their healing programs, begin to feel better, then stop. Before long they have returned to some, or all, of their unhealthy ways. The next thing you hear is they are dead. This is committing suicide with half measures.

The lesson? When you start a program, DON'T STOP until you are healthy! If Greg had given up smoking he might still be around, arteries restored, living into his 80's or 90's.

Stewart

At 65, Stewart had peripheral arterial disease. The circulation to his legs was increasingly restricted, with smoking the prime culprit. Stewart's lower legs were dark mottled red, his feet almost black. Dramatic action was called for. Surprising everyone, Stewart embarked on a 10-day juice fast at our 'Homestay' Retreat. He stopped smoking and each day had 3 sessions of contrast bathing (hydrotherapy) on his legs and feet, juice-fasting, dry skin brushing, sesame oil massage, swimming and walking. When he left you could definitely see an improvement. How much of an improvement became clear, when a few days after finishing his program, Stewart called to say he had just completed an 8km morning walk on the beach. I am used to seeing dramatic improvement but that kind of progress is astonishing.

Stewart was understandably delighted and promised to continue the good work after he left the retreat. Two weeks later, while dropping my adoptive daughter off at school, I spotted him smoking in the street. My heart sank.

"Why, why, why?!"

Why would anyone do this after making such spectacular progress?

I knew the answer. Stewart was bored. He lived alone and old habits die hard. It did not take him long to get back to his cigarette, pals and beer. He convinced himself he would be okay and told me he was still swimming regularly. Two years later Stewart died in intensive care, with half his oesophagus removed, his blackened legs scheduled for amputation and his family £25,000 poorer.

There is one Law you cannot get around. Your body does not care for justifications and delusions. **It only experiences consequences.**

"The art of medicine consists in amusing the patient while nature cures the disease."
*- **Voltaire***

Chapter 8
Nutrition and Healing

Every cell in our body is created from the food we eat, water we drink and air we breathe. The food choices we make influence our mood, energy, appearance, health and wellbeing. Cultures around the world understand. Hippocrates understood. The great healers of the 20th Century understood. The 'Alt-Med' community of today understands. You need to understand, **We Are What We Eat.**

That being so, how is it multinational fast food chains, like McDonald's and Burger King, are permitted to open outlets in top hospitals, including children's hospitals, selling burgers, nuggets and fries? In March 2015, a **UK Parliamentary Committee Report** quoted Prof Theresa Marteau, an expert in public health, at Cambridge University, who said:

"...it is at best anomalous and at worst negligent that NHS properties continue to serve foods high in sugar, fat and salt, as exemplified by McDonald's and Burger King outlets in some of our most prestigious hospitals, including Guy's hospital in London and Addenbrooke's hospital in Cambridge."

A British cardiologist was less diplomatic...

"It is nothing short of obscene that the very institutions that are supposed to be setting an example of good health, our hospitals, have become a branding opportunity for the junk food industry."

"It is perhaps not surprising that 50% of the NHS 1.4 million employees are themselves overweight or obese. Banning the sale of junk food in hospitals is long overdue."

In Australia, The Royal Children's Hospital in Melbourne has a McDonald's operating inside its building. In the U.S. Chick-fil-A has at least 20 hospital locations, McDonald's 18, and Wendy's at least five, according to the **Physicians Committee for Responsible Medicine**. McDonald's delivers meals right to sick patients' beds *(I wonder if that includes the Heart Ward?)*. Hospital food is notoriously poor. You can understand why patients and visitors do not wish to eat it. Elderly patients come out of hospitals more malnourished than when they went in. The rate of malnutrition in hospitals is around 40%.

Many fascinating books and articles have been written about food. The importance of fibre, herbs, vitamins, antioxidants, phytochemicals, enzymes and which food is best for this or that condition. A great book of this type is **'The Rainbow Diet'** by Chris Woollams, who created the **CancerActive** charity and web site, after his daughter died of a brain tumour. Written to help beat cancer it is a 'must read' no matter what disorder you have. Not all books are as well written and researched. Many are written by people who have never healed a patient or tossed a Mediterranean salad. They list what herbs are good for cholesterol, or constipation, and enthuse about 'Superfoods' and raw food. This is fine. Proper nutrition is crucial to health. If you can find untainted food, master the recipes and have the motivation to alter and stick with your diet, there is every chance you will see an improvement in your condition.

A focus on nutrition alone can fail because we are more than the physical body. We are emotional, psychological, energetic and spiritual beings, affected by our outer and inner environment. We can eat the best food and the most potent herbs but if their healing factors cannot get to where they are needed, we see little benefit. If we eat when upset, food becomes toxic. Even when we eat healthily, healing eludes us because our bodies are backed-up, with waste.

Hippocrates, the 'Father of Modern Medicine', said "Let Food Be Thy Medicine"' but he did not live in a time of 'Agri-business', where genetically-modified 'Frankenfood' is grown in soil stripped of vital nutrients and doused with millions of tons of toxic chemicals... herbicides, pesticides, fungicides and 'fertilizers'... turning vast tracts of once-fertile, arable land, into mineral-deficient, 'dead' deserts. He did not live in a time when 70% of the population were obese, their bodies and minds devastated by industrialized oils, fake sugars, msg, trans-fats, preservatives, household cleaning products, insecticides and cosmetics. Seduced into consuming poisons, by deceitful marketing, where 'Diet' and 'Low-Fat' cause sickness and obesity. He did not live in a time when millions of stressed adults and over-stimulated children were turned into 'zombies' by psychiatry and its 'chemical coshes'.

Calling Hippocrates the "Father of Modern Medicine" is classic linking. Hippocrates would **disown** the Doctors of today.

It is impossible to stay healthy, or heal a disorder, on a vegetarian diet, when the commercial vegetables you eat are toxic and deficient. Or a vegan diet, if it is unsuitable for your Constitutional or Metabolic Type. You will make yourself sicker. I know. It happened to me.

"AHAH! HEH HEH HEH HEH! So! You won't take warning, eh? All the worse for you... And now, my beauties - something with poison in it I think. With poison in it! But attractive to the eye!"
- The Wicked Witch of the West, in The Wizard of Oz

Chapter 9
There Is No Food in a Supermarket

"Everyone is eating it, it must be okay"
"Food companies wouldn't harm us. There are laws against it"
"Regulatory bodies protect consumers. It's all tested"
"I am not sick and have been eating this food for years"
"There's no other choice in my area"
"It's cheap and convenient"

What a glittering display lines our supermarket shelves. In the largest stores, you may find 50,000 different products. The choice seems incredible. Most of us shop at the Supermarket, Hyper Market or local Family Mart. I go regularly. Not to buy food but to while away an hour or two, indulging in my favourite pastime, 'people-watching'. My trips are both comedy and tragedy. Comedy, because I sometimes spot friends, or those who have been to see me for advice, racing away from me with half-filled shopping trolleys. Tragedy, because they don't want me to see the 'treats' filling their trolleys. It's no contest. I am built for speed and invariably catch them. Not to wag a disapproving finger but to reassure them it is okay and not to be embarrassed. Rome isn't built in a day and unless you are highly motivated, you cannot switch from an unhealthy lifestyle to a healthy one, overnight. You will find it too stressful and give up.

I am different to friends. Where they see tasty 'food', I see genetically-modified corn, grown in nutritionally-deficient soil, coated in dangerous chemicals, heated, irradiated, re-formed from homogenized gloop into different shapes, mixed with fillers, with added fructose corn syrup (or aspartame), flavourings, colourings, preservatives and any combination of a thousand different chemicals. By the time it emerges from being processed, it has been stripped of live enzymes, natural vitamins and minerals. Some are added back. Only, instead of natural, bio-available nutrients, they add fractions of synthetic chemicals and crushed rocks. Put a picture of alien robots or dancing fruit on the box; complete the illusion it is 'food' by printing '**100% Natural**' and '**Fortified with Vitamins and Minerals!**' and watch it fly off the shelf. We give this to children, when we wouldn't give it to our pets.

Animals aren't confused. They know the garbage we are buying is not food. It may look like food, taste like food, smell like food and they call it food but 'Fido' wouldn't touch it if he was starving. We even tell our children, when they are eating their chips or sodas…*"Don't give that to the dog, it's bad for them"* without a thought it must also be bad for us. Insanity! It is not just insane. When we feed our children foods lacking in nutrition, saturated with sugar, salt and trans-fats, loaded with calories and laced with chemicals and they subsequently suffer cancer, diabetes, obesity and so on, what do we call this? Child abuse? Neglect? Manslaughter? You do not want to hear this because you love your children but if you understand the relationship between diet and sickness yet still give your children these foods, what else do you call it?

Why do we do this to our children and ourselves? It is as if the mind is splintered into separate compartments. One compartment is instinctive. Like the dog, it says, "stay away from this". Another compartment is rational, it knows the food is fattening and toxic and it, too, says, "stay away from this". Another compartment is impressionable. This is the compartment food companies fill with repetitive, comforting, emotional messages which say "Drink me. I will make your bones strong". "Eat me. I am natural and healthy". Children's cereals are a prime example. Looking at one cereal packet recently, I saw the following 'hooks' on the front:

'Simply Nutritious'
'Gluten-Free!'
'No Artificial Colours or Flavours'
'With Whole Grain!'

Encouraging messages, indeed. But hold on. A few are missing:

'High in Poisonous Sugars'
'With added GM FrankenCorn'
'Homogenized and Plasticized'
'Fortified With BHT'

'BHT' is a chemical called Butylated Hydroxytoluene, an endocrine disruptor, linked to cancer in animal studies and banned in Europe. There are far safer additives that do the same job as BHT, yet food giants in the U.S. still use it. With selective messages like this and no mention of the down-side, we are seduced into eating it and guaranteed to keep doing so.

Foods are formulated to stimulate your 'Bliss Point'. This is the exact amount of sugar, salt, fat, etc… that delights the pleasure sensors in your brain. Your resistance weakens and you easily surrender until, months or years later, chronic sickness and/or obesity forces you to wake up from the trance into which you have been placed. These 'foods' hook you like a junkie.

Raw Material

A typical Supermarket meat counter is filled with choice cuts and plump, succulent joints of beef, chicken and pork. How this meat got there is something consumers do not wish think about. Cows, whose evolutionary food is grass, are fed corn, chicken manure or ground-up other cows (known as rendering). 'Mad Cow' disease (BSE) was caused by food scientists turning cows into carnivores. Unlike Hollywood depictions of cute, talking, farm animals, frolicking in green pasture, they weren't fed grass but their own chums.

Animals are injected with bio-engineered growth hormone, antibiotics, water, glucose, stabilizer and preservatives. Beef doesn't seem quite so succulent when you look at it a little closer. Even less so, when you learn how badly animals are treated. Sadistic violence and abuse by workers toward factory-farmed animals is rampant.

50 billion chickens are raised for their meat and eggs, worldwide. For years we have considered chicken the lean, healthy choice. Yet the average fat content of supermarket chickens is 17%. So much for 'low-fat'. These poor birds are confined in a tiny space and engineered to grow so quickly their legs are not strong enough to carry them. When legs break, birds die slowly because they cannot reach food or water, or are trampled to death by other birds. Battery hens never get the chance to see the light of day, or feel the dirt beneath their feet.

Educated consumers, disturbed by factory-farming, have turned toward other sources of meat, unaware similar conditions prevail. Egg-laying hens and roosters, used for breeding, are de-beaked between the ages of one-day and five months. This is to prevent feather-pecking other birds. Likewise, turkeys, pheasant, quail, and guinea fowl. Ducks, too, have their bills removed. "Free-range" chickens and turkeys experience the same barbaric treatment. The inhumane conditions cows, chickens, ducks and pigs suffer is a monstrous crime committed by corporate capitalists. A powerful executive, in an office far removed from farm animals, with a remit to drive down costs and increase profits, has no consideration of animal welfare. To him, or her, animals are not sentient beings but an entry in a balance sheet. **Raw material for the food processing industry.**

Got Milk?

For thousands of years mankind has consumed raw cow's milk. In India, raw milk is used in traditional medicine for healing. Amish people in northern Indiana, who drink raw milk, are virtually free from allergies, although they are also mostly free from vaccines, which cause a higher percentage of allergies in vaccinated populations, than unvaccinated. European Union regulations state all raw milk products are legal and safe for human consumption. Humans were drinking raw milk, long before Louis Pasteur and his 'Germ Theory' came along. Is raw milk dangerous? From 1998-2008, in the U.S., there were no recorded deaths from drinking raw milk. This cuts no ice with governments who have banned its sale on public health grounds. A curious stance when alcohol and cigarettes, killing millions, are allowed. One might think that control is the objective not public health.

Processed milk is not the same as raw. Homogenization alters milk's chemistry, while pasteurization destroys nutrients. Processed milk contains traces of hormones, antibiotics, pesticides and faeces. We are encouraged to drink milk by myths like 'calcium is good for the bones', even though four worldwide epidemiological surveys show nations that consume the most calcium have the highest rates of hip fracture. The cause of osteoporosis is not insufficient calcium but a too-acid diet. All animal products are acid-forming in the body. That acidity has to be neutralized. Unless we balance this, with alkaline foods, the body takes calcium from our bones. The irony is, the milk and dairy you believe is **adding** calcium is, in reality, **depleting** it.

Another bastardization of milk is the addition of sugar. I tasted some store-bought milk recently and spat it out. It was unrecognizable from the milk I drank as a youngster. A pint of 'Gold Top' from the milkman had two inches of cream on the top. What happened to the cream?

In Asia, Africa and many other parts of the world, they do not consume dairy products. It is not a natural part of their diet. However, the height westerners reach encourages parents and governments to give milk to children. In Asia we look like giants. I am 6' and am amazed at how many westerners are taller than me. Look at the Dutch, or should that be look UP at the Dutch? In the last 150 years, the average height of Dutch men has increased by 8". In the U.S. it is 2.7". What is making the Dutch grow so rapidly? Their diet is rich in meat and dairy. Could Monsanto's growth hormone rBGH be responsible?

Milk is designed to turn a 60lb calf into a 2000lb cow. The calf stops drinking its mother's milk between the ages of 6 to eight months. Yet we 'intelligent' humans are drinking milk, throughout our lives. No other mammal does this, which should tell us how unnatural it is.

The Illusion of Choice

When you look down the aisles of a supermarket, you can't fail to be impressed. 30 different cereals, 20 dog foods. Dozens of beans. A bewildering number of detergents. Many different brands. However, what seems to be impressive consumer choice is just an illusion. Just 6 food giants **own almost all the brands**. Many brands are made in the same factory. This is true, also, for organic brands, which we think are independent but have been bought up by food conglomerates, unbeknown to the consumer. Choice? Those 30 different cereals, you see, are made with just four genetically-modified crops. Corn, wheat, oats and soy.

What about supermarket fruits and vegetables? Monoculture farming gives us two varieties of apples, one variety of potato, one variety of carrots. All uniform, bland and tasteless. Not much choice there.

No need to concern yourself with seasons. Fruit and vegetables are available year-round, transported thousands of miles. Apples are gassed with Methylcyclopropene which stops them ripening for 12 months and bananas, for a month. Sulphur Dioxide does the same for grapes. What about freshness? Most supermarket items sit on the shelf, or refrigerator, for months, without spoiling. The preservatives that enable this, we consume. That nice head of Broccoli in the store, won't have any live enzymes, has been grown in nutrient-depleted soil and is saturated with pesticides throughout its growth cycle. Who cares? It resembles broccoli.

Government subsidies to mammoth corporations, who, due to revolving-door politics and campaign contributions, ARE the government, make grains cheaper than fresh fruit and vegetables. This contributes hugely to sickness in society because poor families cannot afford healthier produce and are forced to eat low-cost, inferior-quality food. The Food Industry isn't embarrassed about poor quality. It **tells** us they are feeding us junk. We eat it and eat it, encouraged by a scary-looking clown, a bottle of red ketchup and artificially-coloured, sugar-water, with bubbles.

Prior to the advent of large-scale farming, mankind ate fresh, living produce. Ripe fruit was eaten straight off the tree. Vegetables would be eaten shortly after being harvested, were grown locally and eaten in season. When I eat truly organic fruits and vegetables they are mouth-watering and delicious! Introduce them to someone addicted to junk food and they turn their nose up, or spit them out as 'tasteless'. Recently, I met a young lady with the usual clutch of disorders... obesity, Type II diabetes, high blood pressure, constipation and high cholesterol. *"I don't do vegetables"*, she said, needlessly. Her symptoms made it obvious.

Fructose Corn Syrup

Many people ask me how to get rid of belly fat? In early 2013, I conducted a trial. I have always been slim and struggle to gain weight. One iced-Mocha coffee per day changed that. I never drank coffee in the past because it makes my head spin and keeps me awake. However, there is no denying these fancy coffees smell great and taste delicious. After a few weeks I noticed my waistline thickening. Then realized I was addicted. If I did not get my coffee, I craved it. After 9 months, I switched to iced tea. It didn't help. The waistline kept expanding. Within 18 months I had gone from a 31" waist to 36". I had put on 9kg. My six-pack was now a one-pack. From 1 drink per day, with no sugar.

The culprit was easy to identify, since nothing else in my diet had changed. While I requested "No sugar", vendors were using condensed and evaporated milk. I ignored the evaporated milk, since its sugar content is fairly low, which left the thick condensed stuff. There are 1000 calories in one cup of condensed milk. That is high but I was only getting a teaspoonful, around 100 calories. Insufficient to cause such dramatic weight gain. If it wasn't the calories it must be something else.

Dramatic action was called for. An 8-day, sugar-free, juice-fast, kick-started the reduction of my waistline, purging whatever garbage had built up in my system and ending my cravings. With the help of a diet of reducing foods, within 3 months, my weight had returned to normal.

*[Read the chapter **'The 6 Tastes'** to understand how to end sugar cravings without having to fast].*

What had I learned from my 'research'?

1. Fake sugar is converted to fat.
2. Fat did not cause my weight gain. SUGAR did.
3. The sugar was HIGHLY addictive. This shocked me the most.
4. In a body that struggles to gain weight, the gain was rapid. As if my body did not metabolize the sweetened milk at all. Just plonked it straight into my adipose fat cells.
5. FCS caused severe leg cramps.
6. Cravings for 'sweet' developed, shortly after eating a meal. I became hypoglycemic.
7. The coffee/sugar combination made me jittery and often gave me heartburn. (Coffee is very acid-forming).
8. If this could happen to me, so easily, I now understood why so many are addicted and obese.

Almost certainly the cause of my weight gain was Fructose Corn Syrup (FCS). A chemically-altered sweetener, in widespread use. Why is FCS a problem?

Glucose is a natural sugar, easy to metabolize. Fructose is different. The liver is unable to properly metabolize fructose and stores the excess energy in fat cells, for use later. Over time the liver becomes 'fatty', then the stomach, then the rest of the body. Manufacturers are sensitive about consumers knowing FCS is in condensed milk. FCS is derived from GM corn. Due to subsidies it is cheaper than cane sugar. Food scientists have altered the structure of this compound and will not reveal how they make it. **Dr Mark Hyman**, an American physician, informs us...

'...The average American increased their consumption of HFCS (mostly from sugar sweetened drinks and processed food) from zero to over 60 pounds, per person, per year. During that time period, obesity rates have more than tripled and diabetes incidence has increased more than seven fold.'

In the United States, HFCS has become a sucrose replacement for honey bees. Beekeepers are putting HFCS INSIDE the hives. The collapse of bee colonies has been linked to this dietary change.

The sensible thing to do would be to withdraw HFCS from the market until we know it is safe. Producers think otherwise. Like the Tobacco Industry before it, they leaped into defence mode, with massive misinformation campaigns. Physicians were presented with 'science' showing HFCS was no different to other sugar. Professors of nutrition and experts from Harvard were recruited to spread the message to the public. Millions of dollars were invested.

When you go to your Doctor and say,

"Doctor. I think fructose corn syrup is making me fat. Should I eliminate it from my diet?"

The Doctor will likely repeat industry propaganda,

"Sugar is sugar".

No it isn't.

An alarming side effect was cramp. I would drink a sweetened tea, or coffee, and within an hour, be hit by an excruciating 'charley horse'. The cramp was worst at night. I would fly out of bed, hopping and howling around the bedroom, trying to force my arched foot, flat on the floor, to relieve the painful cramp. Two glasses of hot (not scalding) water would eventually do the trick. At first I did not link the cramps to the coffee, because they also occurred after eating biscuits, then I found FCS is a sweetener in biscuits. Since cutting out biscuits and condensed milk, there has been no more cramp.

Another effect was sugar cravings. 30 minutes after eating, I would feel a powerful craving for something sweet. This was new and troubling. Postprandial (after a meal) hypoglycaemia occurs when your blood sugar levels drop dramatically and the brain says, *"Quick! I need glucose!"* Hypoglycaemia is a prelude to full blown diabetes.

That was it. I ended my addiction/experiment.

Aspartame

Another consumer worry is Aspartame. You may know it as Canderel, Nutrasweet, Equal or Spoonful. If you have not looked at the history of this sweetener, please do. The first thing to understand about Aspartame is it is not a natural sweetener like sugar cane, maple syrup, honey or stevia. It is a synthetic chemical, 200x sweeter than sugar, discovered by accident in 1965. The company that discovered it, G.D. Searle, were refused FDA approval, until 1980, due to concerns about toxicity and brain tumours. However, when senior politician Donald Rumsfeld joined the board, Aspartame gained approval. Aspartame is now in 9000 products, worldwide, including chewing gum, yogurt, diet soft drinks, flavoured sports and energy drinks, fruit-juices, puddings, cereals and powdered beverage mixes. If you eat processed food it is virtually impossible to avoid it.

Why is Aspartame troubling? Every time you take in Aspartame you get a micro-dose of three poisons, two of which are known carcinogens – formaldehyde and formic acid. The third, DKP, is a tumour agent. Aspartame-poisoning causes allergies and sensitivities and mimics diseases and disease syndromes. It is difficult to pin down the exact scale of the problem because most people with health issues will have no idea what is causing their symptoms. The largest numbers of complaints to the U.S. Department of Health are for headache, dizziness, depression, vomiting, abdominal pain/cramps, changes in vision, seizures and memory loss. **Dr Woodrow Monte**, Professor of Food Science and Nutrition at Arizona State University has studied Aspartame for 30 years and established direct links between Aspartame and several diseases, including cancer, heart disease, multiple sclerosis and Alzheimer's. In the UK, a University of Liverpool test-tube study found that, when mixed with a common food colour, aspartame becomes toxic to brain cells. Trials, on rats, caused brain tumours, yet Aspartame was still approved. Rates of brain tumours in children are on the increase.

One sign consumers are wising up to the danger is Pepsi taking Aspartame out of diet soda. However, its replacement, Sucralose, is 600x sweeter than cane sugar. Out of the frying pan and into the fire?

A worrying new development comes from manufacturers seeking to sweeten milk and dairy products with these artificial sugars, without declaring it. If the GM soy milk you are drinking is sweetened with Aspartame and you are sickened by it, you will never know the cause because the ingredients will not be on the label.

Water, Water, Everywhere

Supermarkets provide a one-stop-shop for all our needs. So, you would expect to see water, one of our basic needs, on the shelves. There are all kinds of water on offer. Mineral water, spring water, coloured water, flavoured water, water with bubbles, water from icebergs, kiddies' water.

Once-free natural springs and water supplies have been bought up by giants like Pepsico, Coke and Nestle and sold back to the public. There was controversy in the UK in 2013 when it was discovered 30% of store-bought bottled water came from the tap (around 50% today). Then even more, when it was found bottled water cost more than milk. Insatiable business greed aside, what are the dangers in water? The list of contaminants is long. Fluoride, Chlorine, BPA (bisphenol A) from plastic bottles, endocrine disruptors, oestrogens, petrochemical pollution, micro-organisms, bacteria, farm run-off, chemical spills, pharmaceuticals and raw sewage.

Bottled water can be stored for up to two years, during which time, levels of contaminants leaching from plastic bottles can build up. Sunlight and heat accelerate this process. Switching from bottled to tap water does not eliminate risk. Tap water can contain high levels of:

- Aluminium (implicated in Alzheimer's)
- Lead (reduces intellectual development in children)
- Iron (dangerous for babies and young children)
- Diuron ESK (a pesticide that commonly exceeds safety limits in drinking water)
- Trihalomethanes (linked to cancer and stillbirths)
- E.Coli (a bacteria potentially deadly to babies and the elderly).

Fluoride

Fluoride (hydrofluorosilicic acid), not the natural element of fluoride, is a by-product of the aluminium, fertilizer, steel and nuclear industries. Industrial practices produce millions and millions of gallons of **highly toxic industrial waste**. Because it costs corporations thousands of dollars per ton to neutralize, it became necessary to find a way to dispose of it, cheaply. The good old boys at the **Mellon Institute**, who gave us Tobacco Science, came up with the idea to sell it to the population as a health innovation and dump it into the water supply.

Water fluoridation has been hailed as one of the **"Top 10 public health achievements of the 20th century"** by the U.S. **Center for Disease Control** (CDC) due to the reduction in tooth caries it is credited with *(demonstrating how trustworthy the CDC is)*. Yet World Health Organization data, from December 2014, reveals the countries with the lowest rates of tooth decay do NOT add fluoride to their water supplies. In fact, 97% of Western Europe has rejected water fluoridation. Tooth decay rates have declined in Europe as steeply over the past 50 years as they have in the United States.

"If this stuff gets out into the air, it's a pollutant; if it gets into the river, it's a pollutant; if it gets into the lake, it's a pollutant; but if it goes straight into your drinking water system, it's not a pollutant. That's amazing." — ***Former VP and Senior Chemist at the U.S. Environmental Protection Agency.***

*'Fluoride causes more human cancer, and causes it faster, than any other chemical . . . more people have died in the last 30 years from cancer connected with fluoridation than all the military deaths in the entire history of the United States [...] Fluoride amounts to public murder on a grand scale. It is some of the most conclusive scientific and biological evidence that I have come across in my 50 years in the field of cancer research.' – **Dr. Dean Burk, Congressional Record, 21 July 1976.**

The addition of fluoride to water has always been controversial. It is nothing less than the forced medicalization of the population with a known poison. In supermarket bottled water, labels do not state the concentration of fluoride. Consumers have no way of knowing if limits are exceeded. We are not talking the natural element of fluoride.

A big concern is fluoride accumulation. We absorb fluoride, orally, from bottled and tap water; toothpaste; baby food; anti-depressants; dentistry; antibiotics; and through our skin via baths, showers and swimming. Maximum recommended levels of fluoride for children are exceeded by toothpaste, alone. If you look at toothpaste warning labels (most of us are unaware) you will see,

"If you accidentally swallow more than used for brushing, seek professional help or contact a poison control centre immediately."

Poison control centre? Why are they allowing this to be sold to children? Or ANY biological being?

The WHO informs us fluorosis affects millions of people around the world. In Asia, skeletal fluorosis (too much fluoride) is endemic, known to cause irritable-bowel symptoms and joint pain. High fluoride concentrations in the pineal gland have been associated with early puberty in girls. Fluoride has been found to weaken the immune system and damage kidneys and liver.

At least 50 studies have confirmed fluoride lowers IQ. Anyone taking fluoride-based anti-depressants soon learns about its doping effect on the brain. The Communist Soviet Union added fluoride to water, in concentration camps, to keep prisoners docile.

The prestigious UK medical journal, **'The Lancet'**, is on record saying,

'Neurodevelopmental disabilities, including autism, attention-deficit hyperactivity disorder, dyslexia and other cognitive impairments, affect millions of children worldwide. In 2006, we did a systematic review and identified five industrial chemicals as developmental neurotoxicants:

1. Lead

2. Methyl mercury (common in vaccines)
3. Polychlorinated biphenyls
4. Arsenic
5. Toluene.

*Since 2006, epidemiological studies have documented six additional developmental neurotoxicants – manganese, **fluoride**, chlorpyrifos, dichlorodiphenyltrichloroethane, tetrachloroethylene, and the polybrominated dihenyl ethers. We postulate that **even more neurotoxicants remain undiscovered.**'*

In a 2012 meta-analysis (4), researchers from **Harvard School of Public Health** (HSPH) and **China Medical University** in Shenyang, for the first time combined 27 studies and found strong indications fluoride adversely affects cognitive development in children.

Like calcium in milk being 'good for the bones', fluoride in toothpaste and drinking water, being 'good for your teeth', is a myth. Fluoride also effects sexual sensitivity and performance. My guests, on anti-depressants, commonly report reduced penile sensitivity and an inability to maintain, or even achieve, an erection.

When building your healing program, detoxing fluoride, from body and brain, is a must.

Filtration can help remove most contaminants in water. There are jug filters, counter-top filters and plumbed-in filters. Jug and counter-top filters will remove 95%, while plumbed-in, Reverse Osmosis (RO) filters block virtually all contaminants, although they are not cheap. Take care to clean, or replace, filters, otherwise they lose their effectiveness.

Water distillers provide pure water, with no dissolved minerals. Some professionals are fans of distilled water. Others disagree, believing vital minerals are leached from the body. Isn't this what we want to do? Remove **inorganic** minerals (from dissolved or crushed rocks), that clog up the body's filters and tissues?

Where Does Supermarket Food Come From?

Giant food companies process, package and present most of the food we eat. Where do they source their produce? Traditionally, food came from small, decentralized, family farms. Today, it comes from concentrated, industrial-scale factory farms, requiring few workers.

There is no longer a free market in agriculture. 'Agri-business' rules. Today there is only one buyer and one price. Enormous amounts of waste contaminate local water courses, with harmful levels of nutrients and toxins as well as bacteria, fungi, and viruses. The global takeover of millions of small farms and arguably the whole of agriculture, from seed to plate, by industrial-scale 'Agri-Business' and Food Processors, is a global health disaster, threatening an end to earth's rich food diversity. The suicide rate for American farmers is more than double that of veterans..

Does mankind really benefit from a handful of major corporations, like **Monsanto** and **Cargill**, monopolizing global agriculture and shaping it to their advantage? Their dictatorial control over American farming is a catastrophe.

These two corporations have been labelled the 'thugs of big food'. Monsanto have almost wiped small farmers in America off the map. They have shut down traditional seed cleaners, forced farmers to sell up or transfer their crops to Monsanto's GMO seeds and are buying up seed companies all over the world, leaving farmers with no other choice but to use GMOs.

Monsanto is a chemical company responsible for creating Agent Orange, PCBs, Roundup (glyphosate) and other toxins that now threaten human health and the environment.

To give you an idea of the character of this company, on February 22, 2002, Monsanto was found guilty of poisoning the town of Anniston, Alabama with their PCB factory, then covering it up, for decades. They were convicted of 'negligence, wantonness, suppression of the truth, nuisance, trespass and outrage'.

Cargill touches almost every aspect of our food supply... in their inhumane Confined Animal Feeding Operations (CAFO)...

'animals are crammed by the thousands, or tens of thousands, often unable to breathe fresh air, see the light of day, walk outside, peck at plants or insects, scratch the earth, or eat a blade of grass.'

Robert Martin, Director of the **Pew Commission on Industrial Farm Animal Production** had this to say:

"The present system of producing food animals in the United States is not sustainable and presents an unprecedented level of risk to public health and damage to the environment, as well as unnecessary harm to the animals we raise as food."

The risks he speaks of?

• More antibiotics are given to animals than to humans. Overuse is resulting in bacteria becoming resistant to antibiotics, which is having a serious impact on the treatment of infectious diseases.

• Over-reliance on a single herbicide, glyphosate, is creating 'superweeds'. In 2012, 50% of U.S. farmers reported glyphosate-resistant weeds on their farms. More than 60 million acres. That % has grown since.

Genetically-Modified Food

Imagine a world in which natural seeds are virtually extinct and the only commercial seeds available are genetically modified, patented and owned by one corporation. Wouldn't that corporation have tremendous pricing power and control over every nation? Welcome to why Monsanto is one of the most feared and despised companies on earth.

What is it about GM food that causes so much concern? GM foods have been sold to the public based on five claimed benefits.

1. They were needed to feed the world
2. Have been thoroughly tested and are safe
3. Increase yield
4. Reduce the use of chemicals
5. Can be contained and co-exist with non GM-crops.

All five benefits have been shown to be false. Ask the families of 125,000 Indian farmers who committed suicide, after genetically-modified BT Cotton failed, what they think about increased yields? In 2009 a **Union of Concerned Scientists** report demonstrated, in spite of years of trying, GM crops return fewer bushels than their non-GM counterparts.

Ask those suffering from Chronic Fatigue, MS, Lupus, Allergies, Eczema, ADHD and other conditions, about the safety of GM foods? The number of people reporting to Doctors with these conditions has risen dramatically since the introduction of genetically-modified seeds in the early 1990's. The **American Academy of Environmental Medicine** (AAEM) has called on all physicians to prescribe diets, without GM foods, to all patients. They stated,

"Several animal studies indicate serious health risks associated with GM food" including infertility, immune problems, accelerated aging, insulin regulation and changes in major organs and the gastrointestinal system."

"There is more than a casual association between GM foods and adverse health effects."

Ask the farmers, complaining to Monsanto, about the **failure** of their herbicide to stop weeds, about reduced use of chemicals.

A UK study showed canola cross-pollination occurring as far as 26 km away, driving a coach and horses through the claim GM crops can be contained.

Consumers around the world do not want GM foods until they have been demonstrably shown to be safe. Instead of providing proper safety checks, Monsanto has allegedly tried to force governments to accept GM products, by coercing, infiltrating and paying off government officials around the world. The alleged crimes of Monsanto are worthy of further research.

As far as health is concerned, GM foods can be added to the lengthy list of toxic foods to be eliminated from our diets.

Glyphosate & Health

Glyphosate ('Roundup') is the No.1 herbicide/pesticide used throughout the world, primarily on GM crops. Despite this, few tests have been done to ensure its safety on humans and certainly no long-term studies.

- On June 12th 2013 a laboratory in Germany reported finding traces of glyphosate in the urine of 44% of adults in 18 European countries. Highest concentrations were in 90% of Maltese and 70% of Germans, Poles and Britons.
- More recently, glyphosate traces have been found in breast milk of U.S. women, at levels indicating accumulation in the tissues.
- In a 2015 University of California study, Glyphosate was found in 93% of the 131 urine samples tested at an average level of 3.096 parts per billion (PPB). Children had the highest levels averaging 3.586 PPB.
- In another study (5), German researchers found,

'...chronically ill humans showed significantly higher glyphosate residues in urine than the healthy population. The presence of glyphosate residues in both humans and animals could haul the entire population toward numerous health hazards.'

- In March 2015, The World Health Organization (WHO) shocked the global biotech (GMO) industry by classifying glyphosate as a **"probable human carcinogen"**.
- A 2014 study showed glyphosate is 125x more toxic than regulators stated.

"It is commonly believed Roundup is among the safest pesticides. . . . Despite its reputation, Roundup was by far the most toxic among the herbicides and insecticides tested. This inconsistency between scientific fact and industrial claim may be attributed to huge economic interests, which have been found to falsify health risk assessments and delay

*health policy decisions." – **R. Mesnage et al., Biomed Research International, Volume 2014 (2014) article ID 179691***

Occurrences of leaky gut syndrome, IBD, colitis, celiac disease and other chronic gut conditions have spiked since the onset of 'Roundup-Ready' GMO crops, which reportedly disrupt the balance of gut bacteria. (6)

Gluten-Intolerant?

Gluten in grains has been blamed for many gut disorders, with large numbers believing they are 'gluten-intolerant'. This appears to be yet another industry-encouraged deflection. Intolerance should not happen with hybridization. When sufferers eat grains imported from other countries, or those same grains abroad, they don't get the same reaction. What's going on?

A shocking farming practice, not widely known, has become the norm over the last 15 years, occurring in the few days leading up to harvest. To reduce wear and tear on farming equipment, make harvesting easier and increase yield, wheat crops are drenched in Glyphosate-containing herbicides. How does this increase yield? As the plant dies it releases slightly more seed than it would do normally. Considering the traces of glyphosate being found in chronic disease sufferers, it is not intolerance to gluten we are seeing but intolerance to poison. More studies have been called for to determine why weed-killer is being found in our bodies. For me, the question is less whether glyphosate is in human tissue and more, how do we get it OUT of our bodies?

USDA Organic

I used to scan the Supermarket aisles for organic products. These were always more expensive than their non-organic brethren, yet that did not matter. My health and that of my family were worth it. No longer. The 'USDA Organic' label may have started out well but when Wal-Mart starts getting in on the 'organic' act, you start to question. My suspicion was confirmed when I read Wal-Mart, Safeway and Costco buy 'organic' milk from factory-farms.

Large multinationals ('Big Food') bought up independent 'Organic' brands some time ago. This should not be a problem if they maintain organic standards. However, that is not what has happened. Major corporations have infiltrated the **National Organic Standards Board** (NOSB), the body recommending which substances are allowed and which are prohibited. 'Big Food' is now effectively setting organic standards and seeks to add more and more non-organic and synthetic products to the permitted **National List**. Even allowing hydroponics to be labelled 'organic'. The USDA 'Organic' certification has become just another way to seduce customers into spending more money for something that has little additional value. Inspection and regulation is so lax as to be worthless. Violations go unpunished. Fraudulent 'organic' imports are destroying domestic markets. A good place for consumers to learn more is **The Cornucopia Institute** (found online). Cornucopia keeps scorecards on all the organic providers as well as the performance of the NOSB. Having become wise to research trickery, I take the latest industry propaganda that says, 'Organic is no more healthy than non-organic', with a pinch of Himalayan Sea Salt. Food Corporations idea of 'organic' has rendered the term meaningless but there are still many smaller organic operations who are trustworthy. Personally, I no longer waste money and put my health at risk buying 'USDA Organic'.

Should We Expect More from Food Companies?

Food companies exist to make a profit. Seeking the lowest cost of production while charging the maximum price the market will bear. They also, unfortunately, seek to establish monopolies. *"Competition is a sin"* tycoon JD Rockefeller informs us, establishing a corporate mindset happy to crush competitors and anyone who stands in the way of profits. Nations have been invaded and destroyed, solely for the benefit of 'Vulture Capitalism'. I will spare you the savage history of U.S. capitalism. This short video (<u>7</u>), narrated by John Perkins, who wrote **'Confessions of an Economic Hitman'** is nicely done and explains far better than I.

Corporations seek a competitive edge, constantly looking for new products and ways to improve the old. One major challenge facing food companies is how to increase the shelf-life of food? Rotting produce has to be discarded, which costs the retailer. To reduce wastage manufacturers substitute natural, living, organic food… which degrades… with 'dead', synthetic chemicals, coated in sugar, salt and fat, made to look appealing. A good example is blueberries *(found in cereals and cakes)*. They are made from artificial colours, hydrogenated oils and liquid sugars. The 'blue' in blueberry comes from a petro-chemical-derived colouring. Selections from 14,000 lab-made additives, with names few can pronounce, make food look fresher, more attractive and increase shelf-life.

Two additives you may have come across are called 'FRUIT' and 'VEGETABLES'

Slick marketing persuades us industrialized food is no different to organic. This myth is supported by hired food experts presenting 'Tobacco Science'. The media, long ago, abandoned investigative reporting, and do not challenge industry propaganda, until activists and consumer groups force them to. One fast-food chain in the U.S. called 'Chipotle', seeing an opportunity, is enjoying strong sales. On 27th April 2015, it announced its policy of abandoning genetically-modified ingredients in its food, was complete. Chipotle replaced GMO soybean oil with sunflower oil and is conducting trials to replace fructose corn syrup, in its root beer, with an organic sweetener. They still sell Coca-Cola but at least they are on the right track. The wrong track for some, it seems. Industrial sabotage is suspected as Chipotle products were recently contaminated with E-Coli in 12 States.

There is much more to reflect on, when discussing Supermarket 'food'. Such as frozen foods and pre-prepared meals. Almonds that have been gassed. Fruits that are waxed *(how DO you remove that coating?!)* Many are the ways the industry contaminates our food.

Much of what has been written about is indigestible. It is a disheartening horror show. But I hope you appreciate, **'There is No Food in a Supermarket'**. If you still believe there is, or do not care, I would suggest your chances of recovering from poor health are about zero.

'Green' Advance

There is some good news. If being 'refreshed' with radiation isn't perking up your rotting strawberries, it's recycling to the rescue. 70 million tons of food waste goes into UK landfill sites each year. The good news? Waste that used to be thrown away by supermarkets can now be recycled and turned into a source of profit. Say hello to home recycling composting units. These machines take your kitchen prep scraps, dining room table scraps, bones, uncoated paper/cardboard, and heat it all to 180°F/82°C. This decomposes and deodorizes the mixture, while sterilizing seeds and killing bacteria. The entire process takes less than 24 hours and results in a 90% mass reduction. The dry output can be used as compost, bio-fuel, animal and pet food, while the extracted water can be used in the garden. If you are juicing fruits and vegetables day-in, day-out, as I do, you might enjoy such a machine. Only one snag. Feeding my pets cardboard does not sound like a key selling point!

"I spent 33 years and four months in active military service and during that period I spent most of my time as a high class muscle man for Big Business, for Wall Street and the bankers. In short, I was a racketeer, a gangster for capitalism. I helped make Mexico and especially Tampico safe for American oil interests in 1914. I helped make Haiti and Cuba a decent place for the National City Bank boys to collect revenues in. I helped in the raping of half a dozen Central American republics for the benefit of Wall Street. I helped purify Nicaragua for the International Banking House of Brown Brothers in 1902-1912. I brought light to the Dominican Republic for the American sugar interests in 1916. I helped make Honduras right for the American fruit companies in 1903. In China in 1927 I helped see to it that Standard Oil went on its way unmolested. Looking back on it, I might have given Al Capone a few hints. The best he could do was to operate his racket in three districts. I operated on three continents."

- Smedley D. Butler, *War is a Racket*

"The greatness of a nation and its moral progress can be judged by the way its animals are treated."
- Mahatma Gandhi

Chapter 10
What is Real Food?

What is real food? We have become divorced from our food. Where it comes from, the soil it is grown in, how it is harvested and prepared, even how to cook it. Generations of youngsters have grown up having little experience of real food. Here is what they should know:

- Real vegetables are grown in balanced soil, rich in nutrients, containing all 60 trace minerals the body requires.
- Real fruit is tree-ripened, picked in season and eaten fresh.
- Real food is perfected by nature, safe to eat, tried and tested over thousands of years.
- Real Food can be used to PREVENT and CURE disease.
- Fresh, live, organic food, eaten sensibly, will energize and invigorate, not cause obesity, diabetes, cancer and damaged arteries.
- Real food is organic and uncontaminated.
- Real food has many different varieties.
- Real food perishes within days.
- The soil real food is grown in is allowed to rest and recover and becomes a haven for wildlife.
- Real food comes from animals that eat natural feed, and which roam freely in green pastures.
- Real food TASTES better!

Are you eating REAL food? If not and you wish to prevent or heal disease, it is time you did.

Where to find it?

If you live in the U.S. UK or Europe, chances are you will have organic food growers near you. They may be small organic farms, food cooperatives, local markets or individual smallholders. Prior to the 2008 recession, the organic industry in the UK was worth 1.7 billion pounds. Since then, sales have dropped as consumers have tightened their belts. If you have a patch of land or allotment, you may choose to grow your own food from non-gmo seed, which is the cheapest way to do it.

Chapter 11
Finding the Right Diet

Before you rush out to find fresh, crisp, tree-ripened apples, it is time to take a look at WHAT you should be eating. Modern food production has created a global, integrated food chain where geography and climate no longer matter. You can purchase just about any food, from all parts of the world. This provides amazing choice and introduces us to foods not native to our region.

A crucial consideration, when it comes to what to eat, is our individual need. Not for nothing the saying, *"One man's meat is another man's poison"*. Our bodies used to tell us what we are missing and what we should not be eating but these messages have been drowned out, or fooled, by nutrient-dense and stimulant foods... fast food, sugar, chocolate, alcohol and coffee.

Knowing what to eat is a challenge. Battles rage between celebrity, dietary gurus who are sincere, educated and well-meaning. Do we listen to Dr. Loren Cordain, who penned '**The Paleo Diet**', who says we should get protein from meat? Or T. Colin Campbell, who wrote '**The China Study**', and says we get enough protein from plant food? How do you decide, when both present persuasive arguments?

Should we be on high carb, low-fat (HCLF) or low-carb, high fat (LCHF)? Do we exclude meat, fish, or everything with a face? Are we supposed to eat vegetarian with dairy, vegetarian without, or be 100% vegan? Is that cooked or raw? What percentage of raw? How is it my Chiropractor has a superb physique, looks incredibly healthy and claims he achieves this on a **Fruitarian** diet, yet, when I tried it, I ended up as weak as a kitten and my teeth nearly fell out?

What about a macrobiotic diet? The Japanese do well on it. Should we **Eat Right For Our Blood Type** or be on the **Mediterranean Diet**? Pasta washed down with a couple of glasses of red wine? Surely I should be eating the foods growing in my geographical area, most suited to the climate? Have you tried eating salad, or drinking fruit juices, during a North European or American winter? How can an Eskimo survive on raw, leafy greens? Can he even find them? Do I eat what I was raised on, or is it best to go 'native'? What happens if I move from a cold to a hot country. with totally different cuisines? The choices are bewildering.

What about food for healing? No serious natural healing protocol advises you to cure your disorder with a rump steak, unless it's a black eye. They all say 'BUY A JUICER!!' and 'Get those live, green, healing juices into your bloodstream!' My dog 'Juicefast' agrees. When sick, he goes out and finds leaves and grass. He is after the chlorophyll. We may have forgotten how to heal ourselves but animals know instinctively what to do. Whether it is cows licking clay, monkeys eating leaves to expel worms, or cats eating houseplants. Animals in captivity sicken and die because they are prevented from doing this.

Yet, hold on a minute. In Ayurveda, meat is used to help recover from debilitating illness. I have met those who have healed on a Paleo Diet. My grandmother used to make hearty bone soups to build us up and fortify us against colds and the flu. Chicken and bone soups were a household staple, with pulses, garlic, ginger, onion, potato and vegetables. Bone broths are being touted as healing for the gut.

Today's factory-farmed animals are not as healthy as when grandma was alive and I would be wary of using them for healing. Nonetheless, it is a fact humans have been eating meat, and healing on meat-based diets, for generations. While degenerative diseases didn't start appearing until 150 years ago, around the same time refined grains and vegetable oils were introduced. Every year the Standard American Diet includes more of these foods, increasing obesity and disease. Is meat really to blame?

The use of animals, for fortifying the immune system, or building the emaciated, is not confined to colder, northern countries. In Hong Kong, an elderly Chinese healer, alarmed at my emaciated state, cooked me a soup with black chicken, Chinese herbs and spices. She was adamant, if I did not follow her advice, I would be dead in a year. When I informed her I do not eat meat and was juice-fasting, I was met with a withering look that said,

"Have you completely taken leave of your senses?"

The **British Royal Navy Field Gun** crew are some of the toughest, fittest men in the world. They need a diet that gives them power, endurance and speed. I never saw one eating salad. It was always meat, raw eggs and milk. Yet Olympic champions like Carl Lewis claim their best performances came on a vegan diet. Mixed Martial Arts (MMA) World Champion, **TJ Dillishaw**, is on a **Ketogenic** diet (fat-burning instead of carb-burning) and reports improved strength, speed and endurance. It is too early to observe which diet benefits their long-term health but Carl Lewis reports what I found during my 4 years as a vegan. Feeling lighter (not just in weight terms), and cleaner.

Major studies have been conducted comparing the health of meat-eaters and vegetarians over time. The news is mixed for vegetarians. In Feb 2014 a study (<u>8</u>) of Austrian men came to this startling conclusion:

'Austrian adults who consume a vegetarian diet are less healthy (in terms of cancer, allergies, and mental health disorders), have a lower quality of life, and also require more medical treatment.'

'Studies have shown a vegetarian diet to be associated with a lower incidence of hypertension, cholesterol problems, some chronic degenerative diseases, coronary artery disease, type II diabetes, gallstones, stroke, and certain cancers. A vegetarian diet is characterized by a low consumption of saturated fat and cholesterol, due to a higher intake of fruits, vegetables and whole-grain products.

Overall, vegetarians have a lower body mass index , a higher socioeconomic status, and better health behaviour, i.e. they are more physically active, drink less alcohol, and smoke less. On the other hand, the mental health effects of a vegetarian diet or a Mediterranean diet rich in fruits, vegetables, whole-grain products and fish are divergent. For example, Michalak et al. report that a vegetarian diet is associated with an elevated prevalence of mental disorders. A poor meat intake has been shown to be associated with lower mortality rates and higher life expectancy and a diet which allows small amounts of red meat, fish and dairy products seems to be associated with a reduced risk of coronary heart disease as well as type 2 Diabetes.'

Leaped on by the media, the report was a major shock to the vegetarian and vegan world. Conclusions are difficult to draw, when you consider many adopt healthier diets to resolve existing illness. Did sickness cause the change in diet or did the diet contribute to sickness?

I spent several months in Kerala, a State in the South West of India, which is a vegetarian and vegan food lover's paradise. You would think the Keralan population would be pretty healthy. Yet I was struck by the numbers of overweight people I saw, even in rural villages. Vegetarians and vegans you would expect to be slim. In June 2014, a systematic review, of 142 articles, found hypertension rates across India, including Kerala, running at 25%. The increase coincided with the replacement of natural oils and sugars, with refined.

Our stomach acid is strong enough to even digest bone, allowing our bodies to utilize whatever fuel we provide it. I have met those who thrive on a vegan diet, a vegetarian diet, and diets high in animal products. I have also seen the converse. Over the longer term, food, not suited to our individual constitution, is toxic.

The question of what is the right diet is crucial. The question of what to eat, when sick, is VITAL. Food nourishes and sustains us. Hospitals and Doctors make a grave error not understanding nutrition or the patient. 40% of patients who leave hospitals come out more malnourished than when they went in. Hardly surprising when you see the quality of food provided.

Different foods grow in different geographical regions and various methods of growing, harvesting and preparing food have evolved. In non-industrialized countries, food is largely uncontaminated. In industrialized nations, it may take a little more effort but pure food can be found.

How do you decide what to eat? Some eat to live. Others live to eat. How food looks, tastes, feels ('mouth-feel') and smells is important. Is it light or heavy, warm or cold, oily or dry? Is it emotionally comforting or energising? **'Variety is the spice of life'**. Is your plate interesting and varied or are you eating the same meal every day? Is your meal balanced?

We are mainly made up of water. Like a swimming pool, our body PH needs to be balanced. Neither too acid or alkaline. Around 7.35 (slightly alkaline) is normal. Foods can be either acid-forming or alkaline-forming. When I grew up, a balanced meal was meat and two vegetables. The meat is acid-forming and the vegetables alkaline-forming. Now the vegetables have been replaced by french fries, doused in ketchup and washed down with a chilled soda. All acid-forming. That acidity has to be neutralized to maintain the PH. The body does it by taking calcium from our bones.

Naturopathy considers acidosis (too much acid) a major health problem. I think this is generally true... we eat too much meat and grains (acid-forming) and not enough fruits and vegetables (alkaline-forming)... but, like everything else, it gets complicated. Our bodily fluid has different pH in different organs. Blood ph is stable, while lymph ph can vary. Cancer can create its own acid environment within an alkaline environment. Stomach acid needs to be strong to break down food into absorbable nutrients, yet we weaken it with baking soda. Weak stomach acid reduces our ability to kill bacteria, viruses and other pathogens. Optimizing our digestive 'fire' ('Agni') is an important part of Ayurveda.

Life used to be simple. No longer. Reductionist science means we know more and more about food. We know about vitamins, minerals, phytochemicals and antioxidants. We know about acid/alkaline balance, blood types, metabolic and constitutional types. Yet it seems, 'The more we learn the less we know'. Food scientists and nutritionists make discoveries, only to change their minds a few years later. Like a troupe of French Can-Can dancers, they flit across the stage, flick up their skirts and shout *"Voila!"* Our titillated hearts skip a beat, but once you have seen this merry dance enough times, such 'discoveries' impress us less and less. The public are tired of being told everything is bad for them.

In 1973, the **American Heart Association** recommended limiting egg intake to a maximum of three per week, an idea that was picked up and echoed by health experts. The UK took it further, advising a maximum of two, even though man has been eating eggs for thousands of years. Why? Because 'bad', 'bad', eggs contained artery-clogging cholesterol. Health officials ended up with egg on their chin, when cholesterol in eggs was found to have almost no effect on blood levels of cholesterol. The research group gave government officials a lesson in nutrition,

"Egg is a cheap food that is rich in very high-quality proteins, minerals, folates and B vitamins. Thus it can provide a large quantity of nutrients necessary for optimum development in adolescents."

Small comfort to egg producers who went out of business.

A HUGE dietary change that has almost certainly led to many deaths and diseases is the myth **Saturated Fats = Coronary Heart Disease**. For decades Doctors and the media told us saturated fat was bad for us, spawning the multi-billion dollar, low-fat food industry. Cancer and heart disease have exploded since the switch from butter, lard and natural oils to refined oils, homogenized glop and trans-fats. The anti-saturated fat dogma gave 'Big Food' the perfect excuse to wean us off foods that had sustained us for centuries (portraying them as natural born killers) and move us on to more lucrative, nutrient-deficient, processed products, stuffed with chemicals and cheap fillers. What did manufacturers replace the lost fat with? Sugar.

In March 2014, a **Cambridge University** study was published in the **Annals of Internal Medicine**, called **'Do Saturated Fats Really Cause Heart Disease?'** Data was collected from 72 previously published studies of more than 600,000 people from 18 countries. The conclusion? Saturated fats do not cause coronary disease. The fact mankind has been consuming saturated fats, such as in coconut oil, for thousands of years, without any adverse health effects, seems not to have entered the heads of food scientists or the public. Replacing saturated fats with industrial oils did not **reduce** the risk of heart disease. It **increased** it. What did research say reduced cardiovascular disease? Margaric Acid. Found in dairy fat!

There are plenty of examples of State Health 'Can-Can' girls falling head-first into the orchestra pit but you get the idea. Listening to government advice can make you sick. These defenders of the nation's health appear to be working for corporate food giants and not the public they claim to represent.

Like global warming, the science surrounding food is not 'settled' and is used to confuse instead of enlighten. Arguments still rage today over diet, 100 years after the first diet craze, triggered by Doctor Lulu Hunt Peters **Diet & Health: With Key to the Calories** book, published in 1918. For me, it is better to ignore the 'froth and bubble' of experts trying to make a name for themselves and instead, stick with the wisdom of the ancients, keeping in mind, *'There is nothing new under the sun'*.

A useful way to understand diet remains the classic theory of the "humors" – warm, cold, moist and dry – believed to exist in every substance and organism. Illness was believed to derive from physiological imbalance and a simple, natural diet was the best method to restore it. Spend a month eating only McDonald's and you will quickly understand physiological imbalance.

Healing on a Meat-Based Diet

Is it possible to heal while eating meat? Ideological vegans and those immersed in dogma will recoil in horror, convinced only raw fruits and vegetables can, and should, be used for healing. Blind to the fact some people become extremely sick or do not thrive on raw food. Blind, to the millions who followed the meat-heavy Atkins Diet and were healed of chronic disorders. Failing to consider that in societies that eat meat, people CAN and DO heal from chronic disease.

I applaud vegans ethical stance, however they need to face reality. Few manage to stick to a vegan diet over the long term. Studies report 84% of vegans will return to eating meat. How many of them return, sicker than before, emaciated, mentally disturbed, having aged prematurely? Even worse, how many have suffered for years, trying to fix their cancer, auto-immune and other disorders, encouraged by young, inexperienced vegan 'cheerleaders' who, having completed a two week course which steeps them in the vegan religion, see themselves as virtuous healers, driven to save the planet. These people can do great things but I find their limited education, lack of experience and dogmatic minds, make them less than inspirational teachers. They don't understand about different metabolic or constitutional types. They don't give enough consideration to those who are seriously depleted, seeing them as suffering from 'malabsorption' rather than being on the wrong diet.

Moral questions about animal welfare, aside, I find vegans know little about the 'energetics' or actions of food. They know animal foods are acid-forming, stimulant, and create inflammation in the body, and dairy is mucus-forming. Yes, for water (Kapha) types but not for Vata (Air) types. *(More on Ayurvedic Types, later)*.

These gaps in their knowledge lead them to pressure the malnourished, to "just keep going or" to ramp it up even further by suggesting they fast for 108 days (The Masterfast System) or go on long, mono-fruit diets, which to them is the height of fruitarian achievement, rather than the height of folly.

Whatever happened to our innate common sense? If something isn't working for you, there is NO need to press on and accelerate your own disintegration. It is **unforgivable** to see vulnerable, sick people, dying of starvation, encouraged by a young fanatic consuming a 'mango mountain', then wearing it as a badge of honour. The elderly are NOT as strong as him. People in colder climates cannot do this. These people epitomize the saying,

"In the land of the blind, the one-eyed man is King".

A young woman I spoke to, recently, died weighing only 25kg. In attempting to heal, she refused to nourish her body because it would "feed her parasites". She was adamant all she need do was eat fresh aloe vera and young coconut water, and this would be sufficient to clear pathogens from her body. It wasn't. These foods may be anti-parasitic but they weren't powerful enough for what she needed. They are refrigerant (very cooling to the body) as well as depleting.

"If you don't get some nourishment into your body, you will die."

"No", she replied. *"All I have to do is raise my vibration".*

I pleaded with her to set aside her programming and take some bone broth (meat provides strength). She refused. 6 weeks later she was dead. I have met many like this. Mostly ladies. All amulets, crystals and circle dances. Louise Hay and Deepak Chopra. They buy into the beautiful, cosmic vision we are "beings of light". It is certainly a nice vision, which I teach myself (The **Spiritual/Energy Layer**) but this is only part of who we are. Until such time as you reach a sufficient level of consciousness (almost impossible for western minds), you MUST take care of the 'chariot', your **physical** body.

I have been running fasting retreats, with fruit and vegetable juices, for 15 years, seeing wonderful results. Still, I know raw food and juices are not always appropriate. It is important to identify the Constitutional Type, set of conditions and an individual's ability to undertake a fast before deciding on a program. Fruits and vegetable juices are fantastic for cleansing but are not sufficient for 'tissue-building', long-term. Many people cannot break down vegetable matter, despite the enzymes. For these people, vegetables need to be cooked (not over-cooked).

Digestion also needs to be optimized. Malabsorption can leave us deficient in nutrients. Eating too much or too little. Eating at the wrong times. Eating when stressed, can turn the healthiest meal into toxic matter. Priority needs to be given to repairing a damaged digestive system before adopting a depleting diet.

Jennifer Brents

Jennifer Brents suffered for 17 years with 3 autoimmune conditions. Hashimoto's, Raynard's and Fibromyalgia. Conventional treatment only made her worse. Eventually, Jennifer fired her Doctor and embarked on what was basically an experiment. Knowing little about alternatives, Jennifer tried everything… supplements, herbs, detoxes. Nothing really helped until she switched to a Paleo Diet. Improvement came almost immediately. Part of Jennifer's program included minerals (in the form of sole water), magnesium oil and an adrenal cocktail she made at home, using simple ingredients. She also added fermented vegetables a few months into her diet.

Of all the things Jennifer tried, she feels removing inflammatory foods was the key.

18 months after adopting the Paleo diet Jennifer was completely healed, including her thyroid. Jennifer now spends her time helping and educating others, appearing in the health documentary, '**The Big Secret'**.

"Raw Food Is Driving Me Crazy!"

Does your vegan diet make your anxiety worse or leave you feeling more than a little 'spaced-out'? Have you eaten fresh salad or fruit and felt cold and lacking in energy? There's a reason for this. The 'energetics' of food.

25 years ago, when sick I knew nothing about food. It was just fuel and I'd stick pretty much anything down my throat. Later, I read a raw vegan diet was the optimal way to recover one's health. So, I gave it a shot, spending 4 years doing my best rabbit impression. It seemed to work. I felt cleaner and lighter. But there was a down-side. I became gaunt to the point friends thought I had AIDS. I was pale, permanently cold, mentally 'spaced-out' and lacking in energy. Eventually, I gave up, fearing for my health. 3 years on a vegetarian diet hardly improved matters. I didn't know enough about nutrition, lacked support, couldn't afford, or find, goji berries, or quinoa, or these fad ingredients, and I was light-years from being a whiz in the kitchen. It didn't help that I was surrounded by short, rotund pork eaters, whose bodies looked like the animals they consumed. Not to worry. I was on a spiritual quest as well as a healing journey and like the stubborn Taurean I am, toughed it out. Until the pain in my arthritic knees said "enough is enough" and it was off to India to find authentic healers.

Once I discovered Ayurveda, the ancient, Indian, natural healing system, I realised the serious mistake I had made. According to Ayurveda, my body type (Vata) should have been tucking into cooked, warming, oily, nourishing, grounding food. Light, dry, cooling foods (fruits and salads) were the very opposite of what was needed. I had been right in believing a raw diet was healing but knew nothing about different Body Types and the 'energetics' of food.

In Chapter 12 I write about '**The Six Tastes**'. Food can be sweet, sour, salty, bitter, astringent and pungent. Each 'taste' has numerous actions on our bodies and minds. I explain that foods are heating or cooling; drying or lubricating; building or reducing, and have 'inward', 'outward', 'upward' and 'downward' energies. While I knew things like 'dairy is mucus-forming', I had never heard of these other actions before. I realized the ancients were right. If I eat ginger, my hands and feet become warm (ginger has an outward + heating energy). If I eat a banana, they become cold (bananas have an inward + cooling energy). The reason I had felt so cold on fruit was because almost all fruits have a 'refrigerant' energy.

The energetics of food is a fascinating subject. Turmeric is drying. Gotu Kola will move blood up into the brain. Bitter herbs will thin the blood. It matters. Once you understand food's actions, you can more intelligently use it to heal and avoid spending 7 years failing to thrive, as I did. Need examples? If you are a smoker and have Peripheral Arterial Disease and wish to drive blood down to your legs and feet, recruit ginger or chilli, which is a vasodilator (widens the arteries). Mix horseradish, ginger and mustard powder, stick it in your socks (not against the skin!). If that doesn't get the blood flowing to your feet, nothing will.

If you are a fiery, ginger-haired, freckled Scotsman, with eczema, diarrhoea and heartburn, forget the curries. You are way too 'hot' and need cooling down. Cold showers, salads, and 'refrigerant' foods and drinks will do the trick. If you are overweight, lethargic and tend to retain fluid; spicy and drying foods will increase your metabolism, reduce your weight and increase fluid excretion.

Circulatory disorders kill more people than any other cause, worldwide. So it seems prudent to include warming foods in your diet. Ask **Fauja Singh**, who, at 100 years of age, became the oldest marathon runner in the world. He credits ginger curry, ginger tea, low stress and a vegetarian diet as the secret to his long life.

So what about those vegans who are painfully thin and give veganism a bad name? Or those, struggling, who are advised to just "soldier on"? That, once the body rids itself of all obstructions to healing, and 'inferior tissue', built from animal products, is replaced, their weight will return. Will it? How many long-term vegans look gaunt and unhealthy?

Common sense tells us, putting someone who is elderly, cold, frail and sick on a juice/raw food diet, is asking for trouble. They need hearty hot soup, not cold wheatgrass juice. There is a caveat, which Ayurveda recognizes. Foods can be BALANCED. Combining a 'cooling' food with a 'warming' food will render it neutral. Such as eating banana with ginger.

Is it possible to balance a raw vegan, or largely fruit, diet, so it becomes beneficial for the slimmer body types, in a cold climate? I think it is possible but few people understand how to do it. In any event it seems counter-intuitive to fight against geography, climate and body type.

Juice-fasting and raw vegan foods are the foundation of almost all holistic wellness programs. Retreats are located in hotter climates for a reason. California, Costa Rica, Bali. Mine is in Thailand where the cleansing and healing properties of fruits and green juices can better work their magic. Sipping citrus, grape and young coconut water, while lying on a sun-kissed beach, is idyllic. But in the middle of a North European or U.S. winter? No, thank you.

Ayurveda & Diet

Ayurveda means **'Science of Life'**. It is a 5,000 year old holistic, personalized, traditional, healing system, with over 400,000 registered practitioners in India. Fully supported by the WHO and Indian government. Other traditional healing systems, like Traditional Chinese Medicine (TCM), Thai Traditional Medicine (TTM) and Tibetan Medicine, are all derived from Ayurveda. Ayurveda offers detailed, individualized guidance on food, nutrition and diet, based on Constitutional Type.

[A summary of **Ayurvedic Constitutional Types** can be found in the **Appendix** at the back of the book.]

Dr Richard Schulze, from the **Thomsonian School of Healing**, is adamant the best diet for health is a whole food, vegan diet. From someone who has cured thousands of patients, of the most serious diseases, he would surely know. Yet, I did not thrive on this diet. When I look at him, he is a large-framed, heavy-set man with adequate fat stores. A classic 'Earth' type. Dr Robert Morse is the same. This Type does well on a light vegan diet, since it acts as a counter to their tendency toward heaviness. If Richard was eating heavy, high-calorie foods, he would gain weight quickly. For the obese, this diet is ideal, since it is dominated by 'reducing' foods. However, I am a slim 'Air' type. My frame is small, light and dry. 'Air' types need grounding, warm, heavy, oily foods. Light, cold foods are detrimental to their health. What may be good for Richard Schulze is bad for me and vice-versa.

It is not only your constitutional type that matters. If you have intestinal disease, food sensitivities, or an inflammatory bowel, it is hard to build mass because you may not be absorbing nutrients, no matter which diet you are on. According to the **Kelley Metabolic Diet** (a sophisticated system of identifying the right diet) my type can pretty much eat anything. Except when it comes to healing chronic disease. A lighter, cleansing diet is ok, for a short time. The deciding factor is the strength of the person. If you have little excess fat and are emaciated, you need to balance cleansing with building, so as not to deplete your strength any further.

When considering a juicing or raw food program, assess the ability of the individual to undertake it.

"Your body is a Temple. You cannot build a Temple to last 100 years using inferior materials."
– Paul Keenan

Chapter 12
The Six Tastes

The ancients understood there is more to food than calories, and developed, over time, a sophisticated understanding of the properties and actions of food and how food can be used for prevention and healing. This knowledge has been lost, suppressed, or forgotten, in the West.

A very important property of food is taste and I don't mean just the taste sensation in the mouth. It is probably the most important consideration in deciding what to eat. But what do we really mean by 'taste'? There are 6 tastes in nature:

Sweet

Sour

Salty

Bitter

Astringent

Pungent

Each of these 'tastes' has important effects on our body and mind. The Standard American Diet (SAD) is heavily dominated by three. Sweet, Sour and Salty. Food Corporations know we do not like bitter tastes, so saturate processed food with excess sugar, salt and fat. The other three tastes are essentially missing. Our taste buds have been trained to salivate over these three tastes and reject fresh fruits and vegetables which become 'tasteless'. In fact, if you have tried supermarket fruit, it IS tasteless.

'Sweet' is addictive. Ever tried to eat just one biscuit from a packet? Biscuits are banned from our household since none of us can eat just one. The whole packet is gone in minutes. Manufacturers add appetite stimulants that make you want to eat more. They also use sophisticated tests to identify the 'Bliss Point'. What is the Bliss Point? This is the exact measure of sugar, fat and salt to excite your taste buds and brain. Neither too much, nor too little. Junk food is purposefully designed to stimulate the Bliss Point. Millions are hopelessly addicted to these foods, as a result. How can we break this addiction?

The most important of the 6 tastes is 'Bitter'... Bitter melon, dandelion, bok choy, kale, cabbage, broccoli, water cress, bitter herbs and more. Sour and pungent (spicy) foods have a place but are less important.

What is so important about 'Bitter'?

- Bitter stimulates a sluggish liver and improves detoxification. (Dandelion – very bitter – is a classic liver tonic)
- It eliminates food cravings. **Bitter turns off Sweet!**
- Thins and purifies the blood. It is antibacterial, anti-viral and anti-fungal
- Resets the taste buds
- Reduces fat
- Is a laxative
- Is anti-inflammatory
- Reduces anxiety

You can see how important this taste is. For weight loss, detoxing, health and healing and how, by not including it in our diet, it can lead to a whole heap of dietary trouble. I call the bitters my 'clean-up crew'. I have observed, in the north of Thailand and villages of Southern India, villagers sharing a meal, sitting cross-legged on the floor. They each have a plate, or banana leaf, with meat, fish or rice. Other 'plates' come with a variety of dark green, bitter leaves. Villagers are not so pre-occupied with hygiene (most have no concept) and rely on the protective power of bitters (and hot chillies!) to deal with pathogens. Although physically smaller than their growth-hormone-eating western counterparts, these villagers are strong, slim and can work all day on rice farms under a tropical sun. I do see some smoking and drinking of alcohol and sugary sodas (Thais put sugar in everything), yet the northern village Thais do not put on weight, as their urban counterparts do. The 'bitters' are protecting them. It is only when they abandon protective foods that cancer, heart disease, diabetes and obesity rates accelerate. If you are serious about restoring your health, do two things.

1. Eliminate addictive and inflammatory foods
2. Introduce 'bitter' into your diet

Using the Six Tastes for Healing

I will keep it simple. Most of us are eating too much sweet, sour and salty foods, therefore, it makes sense to **reduce** sweet, sour and salty and **increase** bitter, astringent and pungent.

To a certain extent, natural healing programs do this already. The Gerson Therapy. Our 30 Days to Health, Reverse Diabetes, Life After Cancer and Detox programs. All include green vegetable juices.

In India, Ayurvedic combinations are used for healing diseases such as cancer. In Kerala I sampled one bitter mix and, boy oh boy. No matter how much I knew it was healing, I vomited. Bitter drinks can taste vile to sweetened western palates. The good news is, once your body is cleaned up and taste buds reset, you can tolerate bitters more easily. They can be mixed with sweeter juices, like carrot, apple or beetroot, to make them palatable.

"Just a spoonful of Stevia helps the medicine go down." warbles **Mary Poppins**

Something like that.

Tourist-focused spas and resorts, understandably, can't have their customers emptying the contents of their stomachs into the ornamental gardens, drinking foul-tasting juice combinations. Their creations tend to be coconut, pineapple and mango shakes with a sprig of mint and a mini umbrella. It probably won't heal you but your holiday fare will be tasty.

Keep in mind, it takes **only 4 days** to reset taste buds after cutting out sugars. Bitter foods/juices become easier to take while the sweet foods you were eating before taste awful. Try not to undo this good work by forcing your taste buds to enjoy sweet again!

The Hidden Qualities of Food

If you are unwell and desperately want to feel better, it is understandable you turn to experts. Unfortunately, they present so much complex, confusing and contradictory advice I wouldn't blame you for throwing your hands in the air and following the nearest group of lemmings over a cliff. It is exasperating. My answer is to turn to the ancients, who are not encumbered by the reductionist complexities of 'science'.

While studying Ayurveda, I learned why 4 years on a vegan diet had left me cold, emaciated and without energy. And why the following 3 years, on a vegetarian diet, did the same. The food I was eating was **hindering** my recovery, not **helping** it. **Depressing** my immune system, not **strengthening** it. **Depleting** my resources, not **building** them.

What else did this ancient knowledge teach me? That food has other actions. It can be:

Heating or Cooling

Drying or Lubricating
Building or Reducing

Not only that but foods can move our energy. 'Inward', 'Outward', 'Upward' and 'Downward'.

I had never heard of this but considering it, realized the ancients were right. If I eat ginger, blood flows to my hands and feet (ginger has an outward + heating energy). If I eat a banana, my hands and feet become cold (bananas have an inward + cooling energy).

How is this useful?

If you are a smoker and have **Peripheral Arterial Disease** and need to get blood to your feet, recruit ginger or chilli (a 'vasodilator', which widens the arteries). We have all experienced the heating power of chillies. Mix horseradish, ginger and mustard powder together, stick it in your socks (not against the skin!). If that does not get the blood flowing to your extremities, nothing will. Products, like Capsicum (Chilli) plasters, can be found in most pharmacies. Spas and massage shops have 'heating' balms that draw blood to the surface and induce sweating.

If you are a fiery, ginger-haired, freckled Scotsman with eczema, diarrhoea and heartburn, forget chillies. You are way too 'hot' and need cooling down. Cold showers, salads, dairy and refrigerated foods and drinks can help.

If you are overweight, lethargic and tend to retain fluid; introducing spicy and drying foods such as salads, hot spices and diuretic herbs, is the way to go. They will increase your metabolism, reduce your weight, dry out excess mucus and increase fluid excretion.

Circulatory disorders kill more people than any other cause, worldwide. So, it is not such a bad idea to include heating or warming foods in your diet. Ask Fauja Singh who, at 100, became the oldest marathon runner in the world, what he thinks of ginger? He credits ginger curry, ginger tea, low stress and a vegetarian diet as the secret to his long life.

Vegetarian and Vegan diets are certainly healthy for the right person in the right situation. However, some people do seem to have problems with vegan diets. I met quite a few on my spiritual/health travels who looked emaciated and anaemic. Larger-framed types do well on them but slender 'Air' types, as mentioned previously, need nourishing, building and grounding. A vegan diet is wrong for them. Idealistic vegans will argue strenuously over such a view, believing everyone can be strong and vital on such a diet. However, when you probe, their strong line is usually due to concerns over animal welfare. For those who are overweight or obese, 'reducing' vegan or vegetarian diets is generally recommended.

The question of 'WHAT TO EAT?' for each individual is not yet clear. There is an everyday diet and a diet for healing. Sometimes they can be the same and sometimes not. For chronic disease, a period on a strict healing diet is often a necessity. 'Let food be your medicine and medicine be your food'.

In general, when considering healthy eating, there are certain requirements. Food should be:

1. Uncontaminated
2. Locally grown
3. In season
4. Unprocessed.
5. Nutritionally dense/nourishing.
6. Incorporate all 6 tastes.

We need a diet to maintain health and reverse disorders that takes into account our individual reactions to food. These can determined by tests such as Applied Kinesiology, VEGA testing, the RAST test, the Coca Pulse test or observing our own reactions to food (sneezing, gas, bloating, runny or itchy nose, canker sores, excess mucus and vomiting).

As you are perhaps, painfully, aware, there are all kinds of recommendations as to which diet meets our needs:

- **USDA Food Pyramid**
- **Eat Right 4 Your** (blood) **Type**
- **Metabolic Typing**
- **Ayurvedic Constitutional Type**

The USDA Food Pyramid, heavily influenced by the meat and dairy industry, has long been discredited. Many Americans following it have gained weight and become sick.

A study of the **Blood Type diet,** created by Peter J. D'Adamo, published in Jan 2014, said:

*'...the present study is the first to test the validity of the 'Blood-Type' diet and we showed that adherence to certain diets is associated with some favourable cardio-metabolic disease risk profiles. [...] However, the findings showed that the observed associations were independent of ABO blood group and, therefore, **the findings do not support the 'Blood-Type' diet hypothesis.'***

In other words, if you eat a healthier diet you will benefit. But this has little to do with blood type.

With a claimed success rate of 93% in curing newly-diagnosed cancer and 50%, for those who have undergone conventional treatment, the **Kelley Metabolic Typing Diet** ranks highly on any list of potential cures. Based on answers to approximately 130 questions, this method identifies what metabolic type you are and the right diet for you. **Dr Nicholas Gonzales** conducted a five-year, 500-page case study of Dr William Kelley's cancer patients. The most comprehensive study ever done of an alternative cancer cure. So convinced was Gonzales by Dr Kelley's methods he adopted a modified version of the program for his own patients with advanced and terminal stage cancer. Sadly, the decent and brilliant Dr Gonzalez is one of an alarming rash of holistic Doctors, in the U.S., who have met untimely deaths.

*"Gonzalez has given us convincing evidence that diet and nutrition produce long-term remission in cancer patients almost all of whom were beyond conventional help," - **Harold Ladas, Ph.D., Biologist and former professor, Hunter College**.*

I strongly advise anyone with cancer or concerns about cancer, to investigate Dr Kelley's ideas.

In my experience, the Ayurvedic Constitutional Type system of 'Air', 'Fire', 'Earth' and 'Water' has much going for it, with a far longer track-record. No other system I have tried explains my characteristics as well.

If you need an example of the difference a change in diet can make, look no further than **Novak Djokovic** who, on the 12th July 2015, won the **Wimbledon Tennis Championship**, beating Roger Federer. Novak altered his diet to eliminate gluten products and credits this and other dietary changes for his incredible endurance, vitality and speed.

Doing Battle With Your Food

There are few people who can adopt a raw diet and stick to it, unless in a supportive community. Eating 'rabbit food' or 'bird seed' is unexciting, especially to the elderly. Too many vegan idealists pressure others and defend their own food choices. They turn food, from being a pleasure, into a battle-ground. Isn't there enough conflict in society already? This is not the way to go.

You cannot be conflicted about food. Fears about pesticide contamination, GMO, nutrient density, animal protein, B12, which fats, the cost of eating healthily, and the sometimes ridiculous ingredients and faddish raw combinations people concoct can, pardon the pun, drive you nuts. Some people believe we are most related to fruitarian mammals. I have yet to meet a primate with a blender. Food needs to be eaten in an atmosphere of calm. If you are anxious or agitated about what you, or others, are eating, it WILL affect your digestion. Food is not going to nourish you. Militant vegans should consider the effect their hostility has on themselves and those eating meat and show some tolerance. Berating others, because you think animal-free is the only way, isn't spiritual. It is cult-like behaviour and a form of violence.

If you wish others to adopt your lifestyle, instead of making it an either/or choice, sell the benefits. Encourage meat-eaters to start slowly, perhaps by reducing the amount of meat they eat, or cutting out processed meats. Taking dietary change, step-by-step, increases the likelihood of long-term adoption.

When taking the moral high ground and 'virtue-signalling', it is worth remembering 84% of vegans return to eating meat.

Chapter 13
The Five Layers of Healing

8 Steps To This… 7 Steps To That… 10 Things You Absolutely MUST Do Before… 'How-To' lists are never-ending. I can barely remember 3 steps when someone is giving directions. Nevertheless, having a step-by-step roadmap to healing can be useful.

When trying to understand what may be out of balance in an individual, practitioners have to be like detectives. What is the underlying cause of this person's condition?

A super method exists to help identify where in the body or mind imbalances lie. Enabling us to focus our healing efforts on the RIGHT rather than WRONG area. In the 1980s Dietrich Klinghardt is credited with developing a systematic model called **'The 5 Levels of Healing'**. Based on ancient understandings of Body, Mind, Emotions/Energy, Spirit and Intuition. The idea is that disease or imbalance can occur on any, or all, layers. You may have heard of 'psychosomatic'… the **mind** affecting the **body**. Chronic and degenerative disorders can involve one, or all, layers.

My version of Klinghardt's model is simplified, and based on the Ayurvedic view of an individual. To distinguish between the two, I call them 'Layers' instead of 'Levels'.

1. **Body Layer** - The physical body. Allopathic medicine operates on this level.
2. **Mental Layer** - Thoughts, attitudes and beliefs. Psychiatry operates on this level.
3. **Emotional Layer** - Our feelings, which is also the **Mental Layer**, since feelings are preceded by a thought. Whether we love, hate, laugh, cry, experience regret, guilt or shame.
4. **Energy Layer** - Primarily our autonomic nervous system, which can be upset by trauma, chronic stress and electro-magnetic fields. It includes our 'Aura', a field of energy radiating from each person.
5. **Spiritual Layer** - The connection between you and 'God', whatever your conception of 'god' is. It is the intrinsic part of you that never changes. The observer. The charioteer. The 'Self' or Soul. The part of you that transcends body and mind.

The Spirit Layer is also the area where past lives, generational effects, spirit beings and 'Karma' prevail. Whether you believe in these or not does not matter as far as your healing is concerned. While it helps, it is not mandatory you accept everything you are told. Keep an open mind, apply the program, then you will see.

The western world accepted Body, Mind and Spirit, long before atheistic, mechanistic forces decided to attack religion and 'murder' the Soul. The success of the Merchant Class in moving the masses away from worship of 'God', to worship of the material, has left hundreds of millions with no concept of the Soul, Self or Spirit, beyond worshipping their favourite football team and celebrity 'false gods'. People have been conditioned to look outward for satisfaction and not inward. To gratify the 5 senses. To 'Just Do It'. To not look to the Church 'family' for guidance and wisdom but the corporate or collectivist State. People no longer know themselves. They have lost touch with the 'Self'.

When it comes to approaching the topic of spirituality, people are closed, believing religion is responsible for much of the world's ills. Without considering it is the individuals at the top who hijack and distort religions, for their own nefarious purposes. The usual culprits, power and wealth. People do not distinguish between religion and spirituality. The best alternative practitioners are sensitive to individual feelings on spirituality and use language and techniques that allow them to approach the subject without 'spooking the horses'. Better yet, simply leave the topic alone and allow transformation and spiritual awakening to take place, naturally, as it often does in the course of healing.

Now we have **The Five Layers of Healing** in our toolbag, let's start.

The Geordie 'Guru'

In his late 50's, Ben, from the North-East of England, was (he claimed) a bit of a celebrity Guru, in California. Being English gave him an advantage. Americans love the British accent. He wore a black Fedora hat, an amulet round his neck and talked the Yoga talk. Ben had a relaxed, easy-going 'Geordie' manner and certainly looked the part.

I was pleased to meet Ben, since I saw him as a kindred spirit. Someone who was 'awakened' to higher states of consciousness. Sometimes odd-balls, these people are generally far more interesting than conventional folk trying to hold down a 9-5 job. As I chatted with Ben in my garden, it became clear something wasn't right. While knowledgeable in practical aspects of Yoga, Ben knew very little about health. He seemed not to know what Ayurveda was, despite yoga being an integral part of this ancient system.

Ben looked like a drinker. His weathered face carried all the signs. An admission his girlfriend was an alcoholic made me wonder if Ben was still drinking. When, during the conversation, Ben lit up a cigarette, claims to being a Guru evaporated in a puff of smoke. It was disappointing. Like encountering devout worshippers, for two hours on Sunday, who go home and beat the kids.

It would be unfair to criticize Ben. Any knowledge that helps others is to be commended and I have yet to meet the perfect man or woman. Yoga is a wonderful discipline, especially when used for healing, rather than a workout. Nevertheless, as with so many I encounter in the alternative community, Ben still had work to do. Yoga had not really cured him.

The Gluttonous Priest

Choking with emotion I was captivated by a most wonderful sermon, delivered in a picturesque, English village Church, by a huge, bearded, bear of a man, with shining, visionary eyes. The congregation were all weeping such was the power of this man's message.

"Yes!" We all wanted to be like Jesus.

"Yes!" We were absolved of our sins.

"Yes!" We embraced each other, joyfully, as brothers and sisters.

For a moment, the congregation were transported out of their mundane, stressful existences, to a better place, seated at God's right hand. This inspirational prophet had affected me like no other. His deep, warm, compassionate voice made me feel secure. I was moved. So when he asked my wife and I, to Sunday dinner at his home, we eagerly accepted. "At last", I thought. "Here is someone I can believe in."

Such thoughts evaporated, once we sat down to eat. Bits of half-eaten food and gravy fell and coursed through his beard, as the priest tucked into the Sunday roast. He cleared his plate quickly, polished off the extras, then moved on to his wife's unfinished plate. I looked on in barely-concealed astonishment. I had never met a glutton before. Gluttony is one the Christian Church's **7 Deadly Sins**.

I did not know then but understand now this man of the cloth was under tremendous strain. The effort and desire to 'be like Jesus'. To be whom the congregation wanted him to be. To live in accordance with his own inspirational words. It was all too much. He needed an outlet for his stress. He found it in food.

The Spiritual Seeker

Standing on the platform of an Indian train station, surrounded by thousands of people, I looked toward the approaching train. Suddenly, my eyes were drawn to a bald, white head, bobbing up and down in the crowd, its face turned in my direction. Something told me this individual was going to track me down and sit next to me. Sure enough, five minutes after boarding, a young man, dressed in spiritual garb, came into my carriage. I do not recall his name or even if he gave it.

"Mind if I join you?" he asked.

"Please do." I replied.

With shaven head and eager expression, the young man sat opposite and started to speak. Non-stop, he talked about religious history, philosophy and spiritual practice. His knowledge and grasp of his subject, was incredible. We swept through the countryside, regretfully, missing the sights and sounds of village life, as he spoke. Every now and again, I nodded and smiled but did not interrupt. After three hours, of impressive education, the young man's batteries ran out.

"Goodness", he said. *"I have been talking all this time and you haven't said a word. You seem very calm. Tell me. What do you think the most important spiritual practice is?"*

I paused for a moment, looked him in the eye and said,

"Silence".

It was one of those moments that live long in the memory and I chided myself for being so rude.

"Oh my God", he conceded, embarrassed. *"You are right"*.

Yet his reaction said it all. This man needed to be quiet. To empty a mind, filled to overflowing with facts, leaving no room for self-reflection and the inner work he really needed.

What do these three examples tell us about the **5 Layers of Healing**? First of all, we can clearly identify some of the Layers.

Ben, the 'Guru', had chosen a **physical** path, to wholeness. The gluttonous Priest, a **spiritual** path, to salvation. For the chatty devotee, **knowledge** was his way to 'self-realization'.

I did not spend enough time with each to know, absolutely, but felt Ben needed **Spiritual** power to overcome his addiction to alcohol. The Priest needed to **Mentally** surrender and accept it is impossible for anyone else to 'be like Jesus'. I have seen young Catholic missionaries and trainee priests, suffer breakdowns, attempting to be what they can never be. The Hare Krishna devotee had deeper problems. The **Path of Knowledge** is a legitimate route to 'self-realization'. Academics, intellectuals and thinkers are naturally drawn to this path. However, you could see what he really needed was **Emotional** healing. His eyes were telling me, *'I have all this knowledge. I know all the spiritual practices. Yet I am still suffering. What am I missing?'*

I hope you see how helpful this way of looking at people is. How, by understanding what 'Layer' is involved, we can be better directed toward the root cause of disease.

So much for individual Layers. What about multiple Layers?

Angela

At the age of 12, Angela was a gifted gymnast, physically and mentally operating at optimum performance. Good enough to represent her country at the Olympics. When her parents divorced, Angela fell into a deep depression and started comfort eating. Angela's weight gained, she was constantly fatigued and her gymnastics career was, effectively, finished.

By 24, Angela had seen many doctors and psychiatrists in an attempt to lift her depression. Nothing helped. After meeting and talking with Angela, I had a feeling what was wrong and asked if she had tried the '**Spit Test**'?

The 'Spit Test' is a quack-hunter's dream. The idea is, when you wake in the morning and before you put anything in your mouth, work up some sputum, then spit it into an 8oz glass of water. According to the theory, if you have an overgrowth of Candida (also known as thrush or fungus), the sputum will form 'jellyfish legs' which descend toward the bottom of the glass. These 'legs' are colonies of yeast, clumping together, forming strands. The longer the legs, the more systemic the candida.

Angela was classic for systemic candida overgrowth.
[Please do not rely solely on this test. There are around 80 possible symptoms of yeast infection, which help confirm a diagnosis. Many online sites provide free candida questionnaires].

Learning fungi thrive on sugar, Angela opted for a 10-day, sugar-free juice fast. 10 days is the time needed to kill fungus in the body, if fasting. She could have tried commercial anti-fungals but they carry risk and are not always effective. Angela started on an Apple Cider Vinegar fast. After 4 days, switched to the more palatable Colloidal Silver.

Angela felt even more tired than usual, throughout her fast. With little energy, or desire, to leave her bed. Our retreats offer yoga, meditation, swimming, sauna, massage, health education and more. She wanted none of it. At one point, feeling she wasn't showing commitment, Angela asked if she should get up. I encouraged her to listen to her body and rest.

For ten days Angela rarely left her room, except for an EFT/NLP session to dissolve negative feelings relating to her parent's divorce. It was clear something was happening. White strands of dead fungi were being eliminated via her bowel. This was the cause of Angela's weariness. When fungi in the body start to die, they release toxins into the bloodstream. A variety of symptoms, usually not serious, can manifest. Tiredness is one. This is known as 'die-off'.

By the 11th morning, Angela had completed the program. She was still lethargic and down. Dragging herself out of bed, she needed to get back to normal life and join friends for a holiday in Bali.

Many people who undertake juice fasts feel fantastic around day 5 or 6. This did not happen with Angela. The whole experience had been draining. You could understand her leaving with negative feelings about juice-fasting. I did not expect to hear from her again. Three days later, I received an email. It was Angela.

"I feel amazing", she said.

Angela's depression had lifted. She felt *"totally energized!"* Feeling so well, in fact, she persuaded her friends to join her on a 10-day detox in Bali. then quickly followed that with a 12-day detox, with her grandmother, back in Canada. Last I heard, Angela had a new career selling health supplements.

"Bravo, Angela! You were a star!"

When someone is in a deep depression, they are unable to come out of, more than one Layer is involved. Christian thinking is that chronic depression is a **psychological** problem with a **Spiritual** root. Angela was certainly affected at the **Physical** and **Emotional** levels. Her parents' divorce had depressed her immune system. Side effects of anti-depressants and/or antibiotics may have added to her physical problems, causing dysbiosis (microbial imbalance in the gut), providing an opportunity for Candida to gain a foothold.

I have the utmost admiration for Angela. When the temptation must have been enormous, she stayed strong and never quit.

*'The drug industry controls medical education, medical research,
medical practice and medical law'*
– Andrew Saul

Chapter 14
Breaking the Chains

'Breaking the Chains' is a simple, powerful, visualization exercise used to address the **Emotional** and **Spiritual** Layers.

Our attitudes and behaviour, today, can be unconsciously influenced by past events, sometimes going back generations. If, 100 years ago, a family member was murdered (or committed murder) the effects of that event can be passed down through subsequent generations, affecting our beliefs and perceptions of ourselves, long after the original event. Likewise the death of an infant, war, suicide, etc... Breaking the Chains is used to end such influence. To 'Break the chains that bind us'.

The technique is not limited to historical events. Let's say you have fallen out with a parent and not spoken for years. It may be their fault. It may be yours. You want to resolve the situation but pride, fear or stubbornness prevent you. You may be too angry, or ashamed, to face them. Or you have moved to another locality or country. You think they would never accept an apology, nor offer one. This applies equally to sisters, brothers, grandparents, aunts, uncles and cousins. It doesn't have to stop there. You can expand your list to include a difficult boss, a deceased child or soul-mate you are still grieving over. The brute who violently raped you. The 'friend' who robbed you of your life savings (as happened to me). The ex-wife, husband or partner you are still sore at. The childhood sweetheart who callously dumped you for your best friend. Whoever you have hurt or who has hurt you.

We **MUST** forgive, in order to free ourselves. Yet, many times we cannot. When we think about the people who hurt us, it is still painful. So we cover our hearts in psychological concrete, lock the past away in our mental cellar and ban any mention of their name.

These issues do not always go away. They do affect you and need to be dissolved. Do you really wish to take bitterness or sadness to the grave? In what way is this helpful to you? Do you not realize holding on to pain, fear, anger, shame, remorse and regret, contributes to YOUR poor health and can prevent recovery? Do you not realize that, all the time you are carrying pain, the person you are so upset with is carrying on with their lives, not giving you a second thought? They may not even realize you are upset with them.

The Catholic Church understands the power of the Confessional. Other religions have similar devices. There is no approval or disapproval. No judgment. Only the desire to liberate you from your chains. The cause of your pain may no longer be alive, or accessible. Maybe they and you just cannot face them. **Breaking The Chains** provides an opportunity to face them all. In role play. Getting whatever is upsetting you off your chest.

How does it work?

Visualize the parent, ex-partner, rapist, whoever it is, standing in front of you. Imagine them apologizing to you, giving you their blessing. Whatever it is you need to hear, to set you free. Let your intuition guide you. The imagination is powerful and can, even if you think it cannot, picture them in front of you. Ask a trusted friend, family member, or even a stranger, to play the role of the person you wish to speak to. Or if you feel uncomfortable sharing your deepest feelings with others, take some blank sheets of A4 paper, write down the first letter of the person you have issues with, on each sheet… 'M' for mother, 'F' for father, etc., then spread them around the floor. Go to each in turn and talk to them.

It can be helpful to have someone with experience guide you but if no-one is available, do it yourself. You will soon get the hang of it. Very often people do not know the exact nature of the problem until they start talking. Events we have suppressed can come up once we begin to open up. Have some compassion for the object of your pain or rage. **They may also be suffering** regret, guilt, shame, anger or fear and wish to have **their** pain dissolved but do not know how to go about it.

Once you have liberated yourself, liberate them too. Go and see them and tell them how **Breaking The Chains** freed you. If they reject your approach, that's ok. You have done what you can.

Cynics love to criticize 'mumbo-jumbo' techniques like this but who cares? Your only concern should be did it work for you? If success is down to the 'Placebo Effect', celebrate! If it worked because it was the first time you tried to tackle the issue *(you didn't know you could)*, celebrate! You are free of your chains!

'Breaking the Chains' is a 'must-have' tool for my healing toolbox.

Craig

Craig was a humanitarian worker, carrying out dangerous work in war zones. He had almost lost his life on three occasions. When I met Craig he had been in and out of therapy for five years and was on anti-depressants. As the stress of his job increased, issues he had locked away in his mental cellar started coming to the surface. This is common, with stress. One incident, in particular, was troubling him.

Twenty-three years previously, Craig's one-year-old son had died of bacterial meningitis. Craig watched him die and could do nothing to save him. Being young, he was able to have other children and move on with his life, thinking time had healed the wound. It hadn't. As his workplace stress increased, Craig began to experience profound sadness and turned to alcohol to numb the pain. He lost interest in caring for himself, his diet was poor, he stopped exercising and his weight ballooned. One of the keys to Craig's recovery was Breaking the Chains. Initially, Craig did not have faith in this exercise, in part because he was an introvert and did not look forward to the role play. His first attempt lasted minutes.

"Finished", he said.

"No you haven't. Get back in there", I said, sending him back in the room. I wanted to see signs of emotional release… eyes red from crying, lifted spirits, or peace. Craig's second attempt lasted one and a half hours. When he emerged you could see he had sobbed, uncontrollably. Craig shared his innermost feelings to four key family members, living and deceased, with whom he had unresolved issues. Much to his surprise, the exercise helped him move beyond those issues and put things in perspective.

Why had it worked the second time and not the first? I had Craig imagine his son, aged 5, standing in front of him. Then again, at the age he would be now. To share his hopes and dreams, for his son, and his profound sadness at losing him. To imagine his son responding and forgiving him. Releasing him from guilt or regret. To realize his son would not wish him to live his life with pain but instead live his life in a way that would honour his son's memory. Craig knew he was not directly responsible for his son's death yet, as a father, he was responsible for his health and wellbeing. Many victims of trauma irrationally take on guilt in such circumstances. If the trauma is not fully processed, the guilt will fester and eventually surface in unhealthy ways: Drinking, drugs, violence, insomnia, nightmares, irritability, and so on.

Another key to Craig's recovery was EFT. When Craig began the tapping exercise he had to stop because he became too emotional. After only the second session, the guilt had dissolved. The memory of his son's death would always remain but thanks to these tools, the emotional pain attached to it was gone. Craig put things in perspective. He had four other lovely children who were alive and deserved his full attention and focus. Over the next few days he reached out to all of them and committed to cherishing and loving them and being part of their lives.

Cleaning up Craig's body, the **Physical** Layer, from the effects of alcohol abuse and the sickness-inducing Standard American Diet, was part of his recovery. A cleansing juice fast has a rapid, transformational effect on every level. Through flooding his body with nutrients, along with moderate exercise, Craig felt better, within days. The **Homestay Retreat** isolated Craig from temptation and distraction, while providing 24 hour support. Craig's retreat experience led to the confidence and knowledge he could be the **Master** and not the **Slave** of his cravings. In fact, so pleased was Craig with the outcome, he flew his daughter in, from the U.S., to detox from heroin addiction.

Today, some five years after the end of the program, Craig has healed. He views the program as the turning point in his recovery and identifies the forty-five minute session of EFT tapping as the single exercise that eradicated the irrational guilt over his son.

"Before the session, it was there. After the session, it was gone".

Craig is no longer depressed and on medication. He hasn't had a drink in nearly three years, exercises five or six times per week, eats well and has lost forty pounds. He enjoys his family and has become a healthy part of his children's lives.

Which of Craig's 5 Layers were affected? **Physically,** his diet was poor and he was overweight. **Psychologically,** Craig knew he was harming himself but did not know how to lift his sadness. **Energetically,** his nervous system was over-stimulated and exhausted. **Emotionally,** the memory of past events was painful. Alcoholics usually need Spiritual Power to overcome addiction, which is why Alcoholics Anonymous (AA) makes the **Spiritual** Layer the foundation of their recovery program. However, although drinking heavily, Craig was not an alcoholic. He was able to stop once he had resolved his emotional issues.

Chapter 15
Modern vs Alternative

A Naturopath once took a drop of my live blood and placed it under a Darkfield microscope. Looking at the screen, he made some interesting observations. Firstly, red blood cells are supposed to be circular, separate and bouncing off each other. Many of mine were clumping together. This is called 'platelet aggregation'. Secondly, most of my red blood cells were teardrop-shaped, indicating prolonged stress (nature has a sense of humour). Thirdly, many of my cells were pulsing in their centre. I was told this was a parasite. Finally, white crystals could be seen. The Naturopath pronounced this was my arthritis. It all sounded reasonable to me. Later, I mentioned these findings to a conventional Doctor.

"*Rubbish*", was the verdict.

"*All of it?*" I asked, taken aback.

"*All of it*", he said, emphatically.

This Doctor's arrogant dismissal, far from keeping me in the fold, was the final nail in the coffin of mainstream medicine. If I was suffering a chronic, degenerative disorder and seeking advice on complementary or natural healing methods, the LAST person I would consult with is a conventional medical Doctor. What is the point? It's like asking someone who supports Manchester United football team what they think of Chelsea.

Industrialized, standardized, 'scientific' medicine, **for the masses**, cannot and does not provide holistic, tailored, natural treatments, **to the individual**. They are incompatible.

Modern medicine sees little value, or reward, in 'old' medicine and has replaced the art of healing with 'Standard Practice'. Deviate from this and a doctor can find himself in serious trouble. Patients have to accept some responsibility for this. As long as we remain satisfied with relief and are unwilling to change our ways, the health system is not going to change. Why should it? Corporations' primary concern is profit and they are very successful. The top 5 pharmaceutical companies make more, in one year, than the whole continent of Africa. Profits from disease are stupendous. Profits from no disease?

Arguments online, over Modern vs Alternative, are often brutal, exhausting and irreconcilable. This battle has been going on for a century or more. Defenders of alternatives have a difficult time of it because they are often up against paid, medical 'trolls'. What is a Medical troll? These are people (sometimes whole departments) tasked with patrolling the internet, sitting on health forums, disparaging and discrediting proponents. They 'run interference' on alternative topics, disrupting discourse and discouraging you from trying alternatives.

There is much that is unsatisfactory about Alternative Medicine. 90% of Over-The-Counter (OTC) remedies and supplements are essentially useless. Many alternative therapies will not cure (at least on their own) and much of Alternative Health, like any capitalist enterprise, is built upon exaggerated marketing and deception. However, don't throw the baby out with the bathwater. There are authentic healers out there who know what they are doing. You just haven't encountered them yet.

My approach is not an either/or choice, embracing one method at the expense of others. I use whatever works. If Conventional Medicine works, I use it. Where it doesn't, or may harm me, then I seek natural solutions. If you don't believe natural healing works, without ever having tried It, well... whose fault is that? If you want evidence alternatives work, try it, or do some research. Evidence **does** exist. Just not the kind of evidence demanded by drug companies whose trials are designed to test one drug against one symptom. Natural Healing does not work like that.

Lost and Confused

The practice of modern medicine is complex, with a multitude of specializations. Depending on your health issue, you may see an endocrinologist, cardiologist, neurologist, oncologist, rheumatologist, etc. You are passed from one specialist to another, none of whom may talk to each other and each of whom will have their favourite drugs and treatments. In theory, you can create a multi-disciplinary approach (dare I say 'wholistic'). In practice, this is unlikely to work, since they all still avoid underlying cause. The cocktail of drugs you receive will never have been tested in combination and may increase the likelihood of serious side effects. On that subject, why do they call them 'side effects'? An effect is an effect. What if the side effect is the main effect?

On my first visit to Asia I was shocked by the number of drugs patients are given, at grossly inflated prices, especially in hospitals. GPs and pharmacies dispense antibiotics with abandon. The poorly educated population can't seem to get enough of them. This general lack of knowledge is hardly confined to Thailand, but is troubling.

The problem with the micro-management of disease is you get lost within the specialization. Does recovering one's health really require highly complex specialties? During my time as patient and observer in an Indian 'Nature Cure' Centre, I saw no technology at all. Nor fragmented disciplines.

Scientific language is increasingly being applied to natural and alternative medicine. New terms have arisen such as 'bio-resonance', 'bio-cybernetic medicine' and 'quantum healing'. **German Biological Medicine** has the most advanced concept of natural healing, today.

'German Biological Medicine integrates modern medical science with traditional European natural medicine, with a strong emphasis on homeopathy, biological terrain analysis, understanding the concept of pleomorphism, and integrating the philosophies of Traditional Chinese medicine and Indian Ayurveda medicine. It covers many different forms of natural healing including emphasis on mind/body and spirituality'. - **Simon Yu, MD**

I don't know about you but I was lost at 'biological terrain analysis' and 'pleomorphism'. While the German concept may be the pinnacle of what is available… and I applaud its integrative, holistic approach… most of us do not have access to it, cannot afford it and do not have a cat in hell's chance of understanding it. Why can't these people use plain English? Confusing the patient only makes them dependent.

Healing needs to be simple. If you do not understand what a practitioner is telling you, you are less likely to apply yourself to recovery and are going to experience greater stress. A practitioner has an obligation to ensure a patient knows what is being done to them. You may not care but I want to know what these people are giving me and why?

Those who come to me for advice, leave, knowing exactly what they need to do and why they need to do it. My '**Keenan Biological Medicine**' (just kidding) is my bag of healing tools, using only those methods from Ayurveda, Nature Cure, Yoga, Qigong, EFT and Breaking the Chains that are simple to understand, easy to apply, and effective.

Simple or Complicated

When faced with a huge choice of remedies, which to choose? I find it helpful to imagine a sliding scale measuring from 1 to 10. With 1 being the simplest and 10, the most complex. Water fasting would qualify as a 1, with German Biological Medicine, a 10.

You can imagine academics and intellectuals being drawn to the more complicated methods. Lesser mortals to water fasts. To be fair, we are all a bit sniffy about simple methods. They seem TOO simple.

In 2002 I was suffering arthritis in my knuckles, knees and toes. Like my mother, the prognosis was poor. After 44 days of massage with Sesame oil, a vegetarian diet and two bowel cleanses, my circulation was restored and joints pain-free. (We see these same results in 10 days at our healing retreats). My Ayurvedic Doctor (Vaidya) did not speak a word of English, so I was mercifully spared any medical jargon. On the complexity scale, I would put his methods down as a 4. 'Nature Cure' might be a 2.

'Are you one of the 98% that can cure yourself?' According to the great healers, the answer is an emphatic "Yes!" IF you have the knowledge, are sufficiently motivated, and stop violating the Laws of Nature.

If your condition is not urgent, you have time to investigate the various solutions. Start with simple, before moving up the scale. Cancer patients, told they have only weeks to live, may wish to question on the accuracy of what they are being told, before being rushed into treatment. They almost always have more time than they think. Time that can be spent exploring safer alternatives. Even where a Cancer is not cured, you can stop the cancer growing (angiogenesis). This buys you plenty of time. Some people live the rest of their lives with cancers that are not cured but have stopped growing.

It's our own fault. We are far too easily impressed by the complex and scientific. Experts in white coats, with imposing credentials, can talk at length about the 'Microbiome' and DNA and gene expression and the hypothalamus, and we see them as 'gods' of medicine and wonder at their knowledge. The fact they cannot cure a damn thing doesn't change what is an article of faith, "The Doctor knows best". End of conversation. Except it is not. Despite success with acute and emergency care, our arthritis only gets worse, our cancer keeps coming back and limbs are still being amputated every 5 seconds due to diabetes.

The ancients never talked like this. An apple was an apple. Today, we know its vitamin, mineral and calorie content and its glycemic load. Whether it has saturated fat, cholesterol and sodium and its phyto-nutrient and polyphenol content. That it's a good source of dietary fiber and Vitamin C. Medical reductionists can talk at length about the properties of an apple. Are we any healthier knowing this? No. Because, despite this knowledge, the apple is grown in nutrient-deficient soil, imported, genetically-modified, sprayed with poisons, waxed, probably irradiated and it never ripens or rots. Snow White isn't the only one fed a poisoned apple.

Science has taken a turn to the dark side. Bought and paid for by corporations, who don't give a damn about our health. Their only concern is rigging studies to guarantee their next $billion. Science is a marketing tool for organized crime. Health Pied Pipers, lead 100's of millions down the road to chronic disease hell, with plausible-sounding Tobacco Science.

'Fluoride is good for your teeth'.

'Cholesterol, saturated fat and flying pig flu will kill us all.'

'Industrial food is no different to organic'.

The deceits are endless. If Doctors truly understood how the body works, they would never get sick and it would be a cinch for them to heal. Doctors are in the 'disease-management' business, not curing business, because that's where the money is. So they focus on complicated genetics, which influences 1% of illness, instead of lifestyle, which affects 99%. Genetics is 'hi-tech', sexy and where the grant money is. Nature is 'lo-tech', low paid, low prestige and you can't get a patent for it.

In recent years natural medicine has been walking the same reductionist path. It used to be simple. Now it's maddeningly complex. Everyone is confused about what we can and can't eat; which healing methods are useful and which not; what supplements we should buy and what to avoid; whether it's the thyroid, adrenals, pituitary or backed-up kidneys and what can I take to de-calcify my pineal gland? Everything **causes** everything and everything **cures** everything. Complexity keeps us dependent and the professional class laughing all the way to the bank.

While studying 'Nature Cure' in India, I was struck by the fact there wasn't a white coat or machine in sight. Nothing hi-tech. It was back to basics. Same with the Ayurvedic Clinic, in the Kerala backwaters. I could see all the techie stuff was unnecessary. If you stick to the fundamentals… clean the body, give it the raw materials it needs to repair, move and eliminate stress… the body will heal.

My preference, therefore, is to avoid the mind-numbing complexity of mechanistic, medical reductionism. Macro instead of micro. Gross instead of subtle. Simple instead of complex. Natural and instinctive instead of scientific and mechanistic. If there is something I don't understand or doesn't make sense to me, I refer back to the ancients.

It's not as if we don't know how to approach healing, already.

Keep it simple.

We Live in Interesting Times

There are more out-patient visits to alternative practitioners, today, than to orthodox hospitals. People are increasingly aware of the influence corporations, bureaucracies and unelected Czars, exert over our lives. With the political-corporate 'revolving door' and 'influence-peddling' (bribery) corrupting politics, billionaire money-junkies have a stranglehold on public policy.

The result? In thirty five years of looking, I've never seen or heard of a cure from the 'modern' health system. Sure, no end of dramatic headlines,

'Miraculous!'

'Life-Saving!

'50% Improvement!'

'Dramatic reduction!'

'Cancer Breakthrough!'

Such headlines have been making the news, every month, for decades. The idea is to convince you progress is being made and a cure is 'just around the corner'. Send a few more dollars to your favourite Pink Ribbon Cancer charity, and success is only a matter of time.

"We are fighting this together and we can win!"

Poppycock! All the funds collected for cancer research go on 'admin' costs, or are given to companies to test new drugs. Not promising natural or alternative research. Drugs. Could their motives be any clearer? Tens of billions has been spent on public health and charitable funding, without a single cure for any disease. Yet the merchants of death plead for ever more donations, like professional street beggars. Playing on our emotions with heart-rending stories and emotive images of children, whose hair has fallen out, after being poisoned. They are experts at manipulation. It's obscene to see young children so shamelessly exploited to make more money for their poisoners. Dare to point out this and similar abominations and you are angrily accused of wanting children to die, when the opposite is true. Those, trying to shine a little light into the darkness, care deeply about their fellow human beings. Desperately trying to wake them up from yet another spell that has been cast.

Will there be a new golden age of medicine, where true freedom of choice exists and alternatives are allowed to flourish? If history is any guide, not in my lifetime.

All the more reason to learn how to take care of yourself.

Ordering Pizza in a Chinese Restaurant

We've all experienced it. You aren't feeling well, go to your Doctor and say *"Doctor. I've read garlic [or similar] is good for my condition."* It was a mistake to ask but never mind. If he's typical he will adopt his best headmasterly tone and say something like...

"I'm afraid there are no studies showing it works"

"If you take this it may interfere with your treatment"

"I wouldn't believe everything you read on the internet"

If that hasn't dissuaded you, it's time for the knockout blow,

"If you wish to use alternatives I won't be able to treat you any more".

I'm not talking about all Doctors but you get the idea. What you don't realize is he, or she, doesn't know anything about garlic. It could be exactly what you need but he or she doesn't know that. They know nothing about herbs. What little they know about natural methods won't be positive. A minority may know something but are prevented from prescribing because of the diktat of 'Standard Practice'. Sympathetic doctors are subjected to intense pressure from colleagues and Medical Associations if they stray from the orthodox reservation. Even being ostracized or struck off. A powerful reason not to break ranks.

As the witty Andrew Saul says, asking a medical practitioner about alternative medicine is like going to a Chinese Restaurant and ordering Pizza. The chefs aren't familiar with the ingredients, don't know how to prepare it, it isn't on the menu and you aren't going to get it!

It Doesn't Make Sense

When you think about it, it really doesn't make sense that, in one of the most developed countries in the world, with the best medical facilities and doctors on hand, the state of Public Health is so manifestly poor and getting worse. How could an affluent, forward thinking country, like the U.S., have such high rates of disease that did not exist on this scale a few decades ago? Disorders I never heard of as a child are global epidemics. How did that happen?

Other nations' populations are sickening, as globalization spreads pharmaceutical medicine. The financial cost of widespread chronic disease is unaffordable for Third World countries, while threatening to bankrupt First World nations.

It doesn't make sense to be undergoing heart by-pass operations, stents, removing gall bladders, appendix, tonsils, breasts or kidneys, when changes in lifestyle can prevent it. How many do not survive the trauma of surgery, suffer 'complications' for the rest of their lives, or have to go back for more of the same a few years later, because the underlying cause of their condition was never resolved?

It doesn't make sense to ignore the saturation of our food, air, water and environment with millions of tons of synthetic chemicals and heavy metals, creating a poisoned planet, then accuse CO2, a VITAL nutrient, which **encourages plant growth**, of being a poison that will bring about the end of the world.

It doesn't make sense to support a food system that leaves us fat, malnourished, addicted and sickened, instead of providing uncontaminated food that leaves us healthy in body and mind. It makes no sense at all. Unless you are putting profits before people. Then it makes perfect sense.

From seed to table we have an integrated food chain, designed to generate immense profit at every link in the chain. Traditional agriculture has been usurped by **Agri-business** which has created giant agricultural farms to produce raw materials, on an industrial scale, for the **Food Processing Industry**. The **Chemical Industry** drenches these raw materials (soil, crops, animals and water) in chemicals. **'Big Food'** takes this output, works it into different shapes, plasters it in sugar, fat, salt and more chemicals, with names no-one can understand, puts it in fancy packaging, labels it '100% Natural' and plonks it on supermarket shelves. We eat it, then sicken. Not to worry. **'Big Pharma'**, the last link in the chain, is there to cater to the billions of 'customers' toxic, deficient food creates. Only a Machiavellian mind could conceive of such a system.

In the U.S., Stage I to IV cancer treatment, generates $350,000 to $1.4 million profit, per patient. Doesn't this explain why we have the system we have?

What else doesn't make sense? We are playing Russian roulette. Individual drugs may go through clinical trials but combinations do not. 'Big Pharma' is using the public as unwitting guinea pigs, paying only small fines (in comparison to profits made) in the event of harm.

It makes no sense to spend a trillion dollars constructing an immense 'Security State' to protect us from a handful of deaths from 'terrorism', when millions around the world suffer at the hands of allopathic medicine and **nothing** is done.

It makes no sense to give cancer patients chemotherapy where the known five-year survival rate is 0 and overall success rate barely 2%.

What DOES make sense is:

PROPER NUTRITION
DISEASE PREVENTION
CLEAN FOOD, AIR AND WATER
SAFE HEALING METHODS

"There aren't any", you may hear. Really? 80% of the world does not have modern medicine. Are we expected to believe not one person has been cured of chronic disease using natural or alternative means? Not one arthritic, not one heart disease patient not one diabetic? That any cases were *"spontaneous"* or they *"didn't have the disease in the first place"*?

Having witnessed the success of using natural methods, I look at the efforts of today's Doctors, shaking my head. Anyone with common sense can see we are sick primarily because of what we are putting in our mouths. Yet medical education barely touches nutrition.

The Medical Holocaust

Within conventional medicine there are two major causes of death. Death by drugs, known as an **Adverse Drug Event** (ADE) and Iatrogenesis, which means, 'Any unintended and untoward consequence of well-intended healthcare interventions.'

When a Doctor tends to you, his intervention can induce either a beneficial or harmful change. Most of us believe a Doctor's intervention is going to be beneficial. This may be true for acute and emergency conditions but for chronic degenerative disorders, it is not.

Let's take a look. The 3rd highest cause of death in America today, after heart disease and cancer, is death due to medical error. Between 2004 and 2006 in U.S. hospitals, it is calculated 238,337 died due to medical error. In September 2013, The '**Journal of Patient Safety**' (21) made the following shocking statement:

'...the true number of premature deaths associated with preventable harm to patients was estimated at more than 400,000 per year. Serious harm seems to be 10- to 20-fold more common than lethal harm.'

This is just within hospitals. If you accept these numbers, approximately 28 million people have died, over the last 70 years, due to preventable causes, with 280 million seriously harmed. How many have died across the world?

There is more. The U.S. FDA (Food and Drug Administration) acknowledge 106,000 patients per year die from taking the properly prescribed dose of pharmaceutical drugs. Read that again... the **properly prescribed** dose.

According to one Harvard study, systematic reviews of hospital charts found even properly prescribed drugs (aside from mis-prescribing, overdosing, or self-prescribing) cause about 1.9 million hospitalizations a year. Another 840,000 hospitalized patients are given drugs that cause serious adverse reactions for a total of 2.74 million serious adverse drug reactions. About 128,000 people die from drugs prescribed to them. This makes prescription drugs a major health risk, ranking 4th, with stroke, as a leading cause of death.

The European Commission estimates adverse reactions from prescription drugs cause 200,000 deaths; so together, about 328,000 patients in the U.S. and Europe die from prescription drugs each year. **The FDA does not acknowledge these facts**. This is just the tip of the iceberg. Excluded are those prescribed the wrong drug, not reported at all, or recorded as dying from some other cause. When chemotherapy kills a cancer patient, their death is recorded as due to the cancer and not the chemo. Medical error is not included on death certificates or in rankings of cause of death. Doctors are embarrassed by failures and reluctant to report the mistakes of their colleagues.

Even if you settle for the minimum figure, in the 70 years since WWII, approximately 30 million have died in the United States and Europe. Extrapolate that to the rest of the globe and we are talking tens of millions. Isn't this a holocaust? So, where are the Spielberg movies, the Medical Holocaust Museums, the powerful political lobbies, the jailing of 'deniers', the billions in reparations, the solemn 'never again' vows, the decades-long media focus?

When a plane crashes, killing hundreds of passengers, there are thorough investigations. The Aviation Industry learns from it and changes procedures, improves training, adopts stricter enforcement. In America, the equivalent of 4 Jumbo jets die each week from medical errors and what is the Medical community doing about it?

You have already heard about my mother. A few years ago, my wife's elderly grandmother was feeling a little dizzy. As a precaution, my wife and I encouraged her to go to hospital. She refused, saying,

"I will never come out again".

We insisted, so off she went. She was dead, within two weeks, of hospital-borne infection. Her arms black and blue from clumsy nurses, struggling to find veins.

We naively believed hospitals were where you go to get well. That belief cost our grandmother her life.

"Doctors will have more lives to answer for in the next world than even we Generals."
- Napoleon Bonaparte

Chapter 16
It is Not Your Fault

Do you feel lost? Helpless? Stuck in a rut? Do you blame yourself for your condition? Beat yourself up for not doing anything about it? If you have been struggling with a health challenge and 'tried everything', yet your disease or disorder has failed to improve, you are in good company. Very few of us understand what needs to be done and fewer do it.

Are you waiting until your 'incurable' condition becomes intolerable before you do something?

STOP THIS THINKING IMMEDIATELY

Your disease/disorder is not going to spontaneously resolve. The longer you leave it, the more it will become entrenched and the harder it will be to recover. Your medicine cabinet may be filled with prescription drugs, herbal supplements and 'Miracle' cures none of which helped you. So was mine. Your bookcase may be filled with 'How-To' guides and 'Psychobabble', which made you a bore at the dinner table but didn't cure you. Mine too. You may have spent months or years, trying all sorts of therapies. Likewise. I tried just about everything. Very few people are so fortunate to find that one remedy that might cure them. The 'Magic Bullet' we are so conditioned to expect.Understand. It doesn't matter **how** sick you are, **how** many years you have suffered, **what** Doctors have told you or how **late** in the day it is. There is ALWAYS something you can do.

"It's Too Difficult!"

It is an undeniable fact. Most people, when asked to alter their lifestyle, cannot do it. Here's an encounter I had just last week.

Steve, in his mid-50's, came to me, suffering from debilitating migraines. He had been getting them every 2 to 3 days for the last 15 months. You could see he was fraying at the edges, from lack of sleep. I asked him what he thought was causing them.

"Well. I drink every night and when I reach 3 beers, that's when the migraines start."

I looked at Steve, incredulous. The blindingly obvious thing to do was stop drinking and see if the migraines stopped. But that is not what Steve wanted. He wanted a natural remedy that would allow him to keep drinking. People can't bear the thought they have to give up the 'treat' that is killing them *(that's the nature of addiction)*. Or may be required to do some work. It is all 'too difficult'. Instead, they search for a self-help book or practitioner, who will tell them what they want to hear. It is easy to find practitioners willing to take their money. Is it really so difficult? Think about it. How much time and energy did you spend making yourself sick? Weeks? Months? Years? As a young man, I believed I was indestructible. The pressure I was under built steadily, until, of all things, a spilt pot of paint, tipped me over the edge into tension headaches, chronic anxiety, panic disorder and suicidal thoughts. Reflecting on my lifestyle, it was hardly a surprise. I had spent decades wearing down my nervous system and thrashing my adrenals.

It isn't difficult. Only different. Healing body, soul and mind is a fantastic experience. Many people, who have come through serious illness and recovered, say their sickness was the best thing that ever happened to them. It forced them to look at themselves and alter their sickness-inducing lifestyle. Instead of being constantly tired, depressed, self-absorbed and unhealthy, they become positive, outgoing, joyful and grateful for life.

"It is okay for them but I don't have enough time", you may say.

Really? If you think you do not have time, TURN OFF THE TV. Stay OFF your computer, tablet, Kindle or smart phone, then see how much time you have. Or, take more extreme action, as I did. Resigning my job, saying goodbye to my loved ones and retiring into the 'wilderness' to work on myself. Once you have decided you want to be cured, **give it 100%** and banish all doubts and negativity. With the right healing knowledge and sufficient motivation you CAN get well. The most difficult part is getting started. Then it becomes remarkably easy and you wonder why you hadn't started years before.

What is most exciting... and I have seen it countless times... is that, once you start, you begin to feel better almost immediately, which then motivates you to continue!

What about poor old Steve? It is a fact of life, for some people, changing their ways IS "Too difficult."

Chapter 17
Render Unto Caesar

"Render unto Caesar the things which are Caesar's, and unto God the things that are God's"

You may have heard of this saying. I have tweaked it a little:

"Render unto conventional medicine that which needs conventional, and unto alternatives that which needs alternatives."

There is no need to dogmatically choose one system over another. Depending on the condition, use whatever works. If you want relief go to who provides relief. If a cure, seek healers.

Treatments aren't so bad. They provide relief and allow us to function. Aspects of the health system are impressive. The sophistication and innovation of medical technology and 'tele-medicine' is a marvel. The industry certainly deserves plaudits. What used to take days, or simply wasn't possible prior to the advancement of science, is available to us, in many cases, instantly. Hospitals are filled with gadgets galore, serving a purpose. Although I must confess to needing a week to get over the trauma of an MRI scan. What a racket!

There is a downside. For all our genius, it is results that matter and the statistics are grim. Millions are harmed by aggressive treatments. Deaths so well hidden, the public is blind to the carnage and may even applaud it. A recent visitor to my home thanked the Oncologist who administered the chemotherapy that killed his sister. I don't think I could be as charitable. The cancer specialist almost certainly knew she would die from the treatment. In what way is he, or she, deserving of thanks? Think about it. If I give someone poison, though I may call it *'therapy'*, knowing there is a strong likelihood the person will die from it, should I be thanked or arrested?

According to a 2003 Australian study, **'The Contribution of Cytotoxic Chemotherapy to 5-year Survival in Adult Malignancies'**, the 5yr survival rate of chemotherapy, overall, was just 2.1%. And this was taking the most positive view. Industry defenders do their best to downplay the study and its findings but there is clearly a serious problem with chemotherapy. For too many cancers it does not work and hastens the death of patients. Yet they give the treatment, anyway. In fact Doctors are **forced** to give these treatments before allowing patients to try alternatives. Why? Common sense says safer therapies should be attempted **before** aggressive interventions.

Physicians in other nations regard American cancer therapy as extraordinarily aggressive, using surgery, chemotherapy, and radiation therapy far more extensively than the evidence warrants. There are wide variations in treatments not only within the U.S. but between nations.

*[***Note: There ARE a few Cancers for which chemotherapy has shown benefit and there may have been advances since the 2003 study was conducted. Please research this carefully. 'CANCERactive' is a UK-based non-profit, Cancer Charity concerned solely with the provision of information about Cancer. Their web site is packed with the latest information].*

Why are natural healers in the U.S. who have success with cancer, brutalized, threatened, imprisoned (some dying in suspicious circumstances), instead of being celebrated? When you research how the American AMA and FDA persecuted Dr Max Gerson, Harry Hoxsey, Royal Raymond Rife, Rene Caisse, Dr Richard Schulze, and many more, you will be shocked. An excellent documentary (9), '**How Healing Becomes a Crime**' examines the Hoxsey cure and exposes the health politics involved. Mildred Nelson, a nurse who worked for Harold Hoxsey, took the Hoxsey formula to Mexico and set up the first cancer clinic there, has been helping cancer patients for over 40 years and reports an 80% cure rate.

"You wouldn't believe how many FDA officials or relatives or acquaintances of FDA officials come to see me as patients in Hanover. You wouldn't believe this, or directors of the American Medical Association (AMA), or American Cancer Association, or the presidents of orthodox cancer institutes. That's the fact."- **Dr. Hans Nieper, President, German Society of Oncology**

What other extraordinarily aggressive treatments exist?

How many HIV-positive patients would have lived had they not taken AZT? The drug made millions for the drug company... the gay community clamoured for it, yet the manufacturer's own documents show AZT was ineffective and highly toxic. Tom Hanks failed to mention this in the AIDS-propaganda movie '**Philadelphia**'.

Ask yourself...

• Is it true, for all these 'incurable' diseases, there is not a cure to be found anywhere on this earth?

- Is Mother Nature so cruel she would deny us the ability to heal?
- Is health as complicated as we've been conditioned to believe?
- Is it right that only officially-sanctioned, 'qualified' professionals can tend to the sick or use the word 'cure'?
- Do you believe we cannot heal ourselves?

My answer is an emphatic "NO".

Despite their abilities, Doctors are not 'gods' to be revered. They have the same human weakness as the rest of us and are just as susceptible to control and influence. Possibly more so, since their egos convince them they would spot deception if they encountered it. Pharmaceutical companies and medical bodies understand this and direct a large amount of their effort toward persuasion. Sophisticated marketing, manipulation of data, suppression of negative findings, ongoing education by pharma-controlled medical journals and recruitment of 'lead Doctors', encourages practicing GPs to prescribe medicine in a particular way. Do you really think it a coincidence the treatment you receive always involves a pharmaceutical drug?

What about all those studies 'proving' these interventions are beneficial? Peer-reviewed studies. Randomized-controlled trials. 'Double-blind' this and 'placebo' that. "Abracadabra!" the Industry magicians and their media handmaidens cry. The public applauds, not realizing most published studies are not worth the paper they are written on. Only 15% of 'scientific' medicine has ever been tested. **Randomized Controlled Trials (RCTs)** did not exist until relatively recently. The industry is not going to spend billions submitting 100 years of prior medical practice to trials.

On April 2016, the **Lancet**, a highly respected **British Medical Journal**, published an article saying:

*'The case against science is straightforward: much of the scientific literature, perhaps half, may simply be untrue. Afflicted by studies with small sample sizes, tiny effects, invalid exploratory analyses, and flagrant conflicts of interest, together with an obsession for pursuing fashionable trends of dubious importance, **science has taken a turn towards darkness.'***

Pubmed is an online database housing thousands of research articles. In 2005 it published an article by **John P. A. Ioannidis** called **'Why Most Published Research Findings Are False'**. It is the most popular article ever published on Pubmed. The headline says it all. Over a 20 year period, it was discovered NONE of the 'breakthroughs' the media sensationally publicize, came to anything. Most research findings were unable to be replicated.

What does this mean? Science cannot be trusted. Results can be manipulated, or research frameworks designed to achieve a desired outcome. Doctors or scientists may be trying to make a name for themselves. Or are pitching for research funding by placing positive articles in the media. Health corporations may be rigging studies. Just look at what happened with Global Warming. $billions in grant money available to those who find FOR warming, while NO money for those who find against. Is it any surprise studies always FIND warming? Do you think the same 'greasing of the wheels' doesn't happen in other industries?

Need evidence HIV=AIDS? High Cholesterol=Heart Disease? No problem. Splash a little grant money around. But only to scientists who find FOR your hypothesis. As far as I am aware NO live virus has EVER been found in an AIDS patient. What viral infection in history waits 10-15 years before it affects you? There are many unsatisfactory aspects to the AIDS hypothesis. Personally, I am in no doubt it's a hoax. Yes, people can die from a depressed immune system but there are many things that depress the immune system. In virology, the presence of antibodies was evidence a virus had been **defeated**. Yet, AIDS theory turns that on its head and says antibodies are evidence a virus is **present**. When you dig deeper you see the 'AIDS patients' who die, are those who have taken the medicines.

There is SO much deceit, in and outside of medicine, I simply do not trust what I am told. How many media health campaigns are backed by independent, verifiable science? The 2009 'swine flu' was going to 'kill millions' if we didn't get our shots. Doctors outdid each other to frighten the public. I am just a layman yet could see clearly the 'pandemic' was a fraud. Millions of others sensed it too, despite establishment fear-mongering. Why did leading Doctors recommend an untested, unproven vaccine, containing dangerous ingredients, for what was a mild seasonal flu?

It isn't difficult to manipulate Doctors.

- If WE can be driven by mass media, medical journals, tainted studies, lead doctors and corporate-bought politicians, to believe in a bogus pandemic, so too can Doctors.
- If WE can be lured by inducements, promotions, kickbacks, or seminars in the Bahamas, so too can Doctors.

- If WE are fearful of 'rocking the boat', being struck off, ostracized by our colleagues, stripped of research grants and perks, or left unable to pay off large debts incurred acquiring our gold-plated medical education, so too are Doctors.

It is very difficult to be a maverick when the bills have to be paid. Why make life difficult for yourself? The rewards for conforming are good, while the penalties for non-compliance can be severe. Because of this system of persuasion and coercion, you will rarely encounter a free-thinking, independent GP, able to dispense medicine in a way he sees fit. Not in the western medical model.

You may believe there is nothing sinister in Doctors having to conform. How else can you deliver health-care to hundreds of millions of people, without some degree of control and standardization? If every Doctor adopted alternative methods, tailored for each individual, hospitals and surgeries would grind to a halt. Already under significant pressure, they would not have the time, or resources, to provide such a service, even if patients were prepared to alter their lifestyles, which most are not. Yet, this is exactly what is needed, because industrialized medicine CANNOT cure chronic and degenerative disorders.

Another example of dubious 'health' recommendations, which to natural healers, is positively medieval, is the removal of women's breasts and/or ovaries, as a **'precaution against cancer'**. With no symptoms whatsoever, only fear of the possibility of breast cancer, women are having their bodies mutilated. Can you envisage a young woman, in her prime, being given this advice, perhaps because a mother or sister, or both, died of breast cancer? Will her man really stand by her? Can she ever go to the beach again? Are there really no alternatives? How many women commit suicide after mastectomies? It happens.

This is a topical issue since Hollywood actress, **Angelina Jolie**, purportedly at high risk, ably assisted by the corporate mass media, recently encouraged women to have expensive tests and their breasts removed, despite having no symptoms of ill health whatsoever. This was a huge global human interest story *(marketing effort)* and a sign of things to come with genetic testing. What happens if the public learn the risks were exaggerated? That the breast cancer test she relied on is unreliable or that a negative finding can sometimes be a positive sign? That removing her breasts may still not save her? That even if the risks were accurately stated, strategies exist, to reduce risk substantially, or even cure any cancer that develops? Genetic susceptibility does not guarantee sickness. The science of **Epigenetics** tells us gene expression can be changed. Will Angelina Jolie be re-presented to the world, with the same massive media exposure, making an unreserved apology to those women frightened into following her example? Unlikely.

I do not know what you think of Angelina. My heart goes out to her. It certainly does not go out to calculating health corporation executives, signing up celebrities to foist ever more tests, 'wonder' drugs and treatments on the public. This one at $4000 a pop.

"It is simply no longer possible to believe much of the clinical research that is published, or to rely on the judgment of trusted physicians or authoritative medical guidelines. I take no pleasure in this conclusion, which I reached slowly and reluctantly over my two decades as an editor of The New England Journal of Medicine."
- Dr. Marcia Angell, physician and Editor-in-Chief (NEMJ)

Sarah

Sarah, 35, was still young when she discovered two lumps in her breast. After taking medical advice, she underwent a double mastectomy and radiation. Post-conventional treatment, she went to see one of the top alternative cancer specialists in the country, who provided her with a 40-page Cancer Recovery program. Sarah, understandably, wanted to make sure she was clear of any remaining cancer. The alternative specialist was engaging and knowledgeable but the document he gave her was an unmitigated disaster. A rambling, complex (he is an academic) political diatribe; so badly laid out it was impossible to read. I struggled through 12 pages before I put it down, appalled. No patient should be given such a document.

The seriously ill are under tremendous strain, even if they present as cool, calm and collected. They need simple, easy to follow, instructions. The specialist had thrown the kitchen-sink at her, putting her on 60 supplements, not including other therapies. In his defence, the Cancer patients he sees have already undergone conventional treatment, so it is much harder to bring about recovery. Sarah had been weakened by radiation and surgery. Her lymph nodes, which channel metabolic and other wastes away from the breast, had been removed. It is a testament to Sarah's bright spirit and the support of those close to her, she is holding up as well as she is.

Are 60 different supplements necessary? Since no-one knows precisely what Sarah may be deficient in, providing everything, makes sense. However, to me, fresh, 'live' food is always better than 'dead' supplements and obviously more affordable. When Sarah signed up for a **'Life After Cancer'** retreat I asked if she had noticed any benefit from taking them?

"No", came the answer. She took no more.

What Sarah needed most was emotional healing. She had been through a terribly wounding ordeal. Grief for her lost breasts and fear the cancer may return kept her awake at night. Following the retreat, Sarah opted for health coaching. This created much-needed focus for her and stopped her bouncing from therapy to therapy. She has made good progress.

During her healing journey Sarah learned a great deal. So much so, she left London and is now involved in running retreats in Spain.

Chapter 18
Nature's Laws

**Whatever you are doing that is making you sick,
STOP DOING IT!**

While in India, I was taken to see a famous Swami (holy man), who lived on the grounds of a wealthy lawyer's property. The Swami listened patiently for an hour as I related my tale of stress, marital and health woe. Finished, I waited patiently for his profound advice. Drawn, perhaps, from the Gita, Upanishads or Vedas. He looked at me and said,

"Stop it".

I waited, expectantly, for more wisdom to pour forth. He turned away. Not for the first time, I was disappointed. Today, I have come to realize this man was giving me the **First Rule of Health**.

Which of these sounds familiar?

"I know junk food is making me ill but I <u>love</u> it".
"I <u>need</u> my cigarette/chocolate/beer/coffee/computer games/FaceTube, to help me relax".
"What they show on TV <u>makes</u> me so angry/worried/sad"
"I <u>know</u> I should exercise more but…"
"I really <u>should</u> be more positive but…"

You get the idea. Most of us know already what is making us sick. The answer, as the Swami pointed out, is to *"Stop it!"*
STOP eating garbage, drinking and staying up too late
STOP watching TV if it disturbs you
STOP being a couch-potato, negative or arguing with others
STOP whatever you are doing that is making you sick!
Only when you **STOP** building disease can you **START** to build health.

Ayurveda has two inescapable laws. The Laws of **Similars** and **Opposites**. Let's see how they work…

Similars
If I am fat and eat fattening food, I will become fatter.

If I am slim and eat slimming foods, I will become slimmer.
If I am cold and eat cooling foods, I will feel colder.
If I am hot and eat heating foods, I will become hotter.
If I am dry and eat drying foods, I will become drier.
If I am wet and eat watery foods, I will become wetter.
If I am depressed and think negative, I will be more depressed.

Opposites

If I am fat and eat <u>reducing</u> foods, I will become slimmer.
If I am slim and eat <u>fattening</u> foods, I will become fatter.
If I am cold and eat <u>heating</u> foods, I will feel warmer.
If I am hot and eat <u>cooling</u> foods, I will become cooler.
If I am dry and eat <u>watery</u> foods, I will become wetter.
If I am wet and eat <u>drying</u> foods, I will become drier.
If I am depressed and think positive, I will become happier
.

Welcome to the **Second Rule of Health**.

Whatever you are doing that is making you sick, DO THE OPPOSITE!

Healing, generally, requires 5 steps: 1. **First and Second Rules of Health.** 3. **Ensure** channels of elimination – kidneys, lungs, skin and colon are working optimally. 4. **Clear** body, mind, emotions, energy system and 'Spirit', of toxicity, stagnation, constrictions and blockages and bring them back into balance. 5. **Provide** the body with the raw materials (nutrients) it needs.

What are 'toxins'? The **Nemours Foundation** says:

"A toxin is a chemical or poison that is known to have harmful effects on the body. Toxins can come from food or water, from chemicals used to grow or prepare food, and even from the air we breathe. Our bodies process those toxins through organs like the liver and kidneys and eliminate them in the form of sweat, urine, and faeces."

Toxins include by-products of poor digestion, metabolic waste, drugs, poisons, plastics, heavy metals, hormones, parasites, viruses, bacteria and fungi. Holistic systems also address toxic thoughts, emotional, spiritual and energetic blockages. A colonic in your local spa doesn't cut it.

Nutrients IN. Waste OUT. The circulatory system delivers nutrients to cells, while the lymphatic system eliminates waste.

If your colon, arteries, liver and tissues are backed-up with waste, disease can arise. Waste matter not quickly cleared from cells can end up lodged in the micro-capillaries and deeper tissues. Ayurveda calls this waste matter 'Ama'. Once you have eliminated waste and cleared blockages, you need nutrients. These include minerals, vitamins, enzymes, amino acids, antioxidants, fats and oils.

The 5 steps form the core of healing programs the world over. Where differences exist, is in methods, quantities and supplements used. You can clear the body by water fasting, colonics, juice fasting, raw food and vegetarian diets, exercise, steam therapy, liver, kidney and gall bladder flushes, skin brushing, massage and appropriate herbs and supplements.

Probiotics and live enzymes are helpful in gobbling up 'bad' bacteria and rogue cells. Most of us have poor digestion due to the lack of live enzymes in our food. Cooking and chlorine in water destroys them. Gut bacteria, 80% of which forms our immune system, is unbalanced by antibiotics in meat and farmed fish, and too readily dispensed by Doctors who don't realize the long-term effect on immune function. With gut flora weakened and no live enzymes, cancer and other diseases can develop.

Another crucial area is oxygen. Due to excessive stress our lungs are stiff and frozen. We do not breathe adequately, utilizing only the top 1/3rd of our lungs. Neither taking in adequate oxygen, nor fully expelling carbon dioxide. This results in high carbon dioxide levels and low oxygenation. Cancer thrives in such an environment. Increasing oxygen levels is an important part of holistic programs. If you are practicing yoga and not including breathing (Pranayama) ask for it to be included or change your class.

It is commonly observed, those who succumb to cancer, do so after a major traumatic event or long period of stress. Holistic healing programs restore emotional balance (the **Emotional** Layer in the 5 Layers of Healing).

"If I had cancer, I would put a tube in my mouth from a juicer and leave the machine running"
*- **Dr Richard Schulze***

Chapter 19
Curing a 'Great Great'

Dr Bernard Jensen, one of the 'great greats' of natural healing, who had written over 50 health books and treated royalty and nobility the world over. Versed in a wide variety of healing disciplines, including nutrition, bowel care, hydrotherapy, fasting, reflexology, polarity, glandular balancing, sanatorium work, homeopathy, herbalism, diets, acupuncture, craniopathy and personology *(a new one to me!)*, Bernard Jensen was knighted for his work.

So how did Bernard end up, at 85 years of age, weighing 76lbs, on a morphine drip, dying of late-stage prostate cancer, metastasized to the bone? Perhaps because his lifestyle involved a lot of airline travel, long hours, restaurant food and disrupted sleep. Whatever the reason, he was given only days to live by conventional medicine. Until Dr Michael O'Brien was called in.

Bernard Jensen wrote the book on bowels, yet had not had a bowel movement in 15 days due to the medicines he was given (orthodox medicines slow the transit time of waste through the bowels, causing putrefaction). Dr O'Brian realized, although Bernard had fasted and tried various strategies to beat his cancer, he was lacking in two important elements, probiotics and enzymes. O'Brian gave Jensen oil enemas to move the bowels and large doses of probiotics and proteolytic enzymes. By the third week Bernard was conducting business over the phone. Within 8 weeks, Jensen was declared cancer-free and back to normal. It was a stunning turnaround and dramatic demonstration of natural approaches ability to cure.

That was not the end of the Jensen story. Shortly after reversing his cancer, Bernard had the misfortune to be involved in a road accident and was paralyzed from the waist down. The Doctors said he would never recover. Again, they were wrong. The same treatment was applied, with the same stunning result.

Within weeks Bernard was walking again.

Chapter 20
A White Coat Has Magical Powers

Doctors have an impressive ability to direct us and we unquestioningly obey. Public faith in the medical profession, although weakening, is still strong. We admire doctors' technical knowledge, cool professionalism and confidence. Doctors ooze authority.

How can our faith in Doctors be justified in the face of so much failure? Why do we so readily accept the labels Doctors give our conditions, which lock us into their narrow and inadequate treatments?

Diagnosis is the foundation of modern medicine, yet I read anything from 20%-70% of diagnoses are wrong. A systematic review, published in the **British Medical Journal** in July 2012, stated 40,500 patients, in America, die annually in Intensive Care Units because of misdiagnosis. That is the same as die from breast cancer. Have you seen any charitable drives seeking funds to end misdiagnosis?

Not so long ago doctors in America were recommending smoking as being 'Good for the Brain'. Today, they couldn't get away with such a claim. Or could they? Lead doctors (opinion-formers) promote similar myths on behalf of their corporate sponsors. There are countless examples. One is "High Cholesterol causes or contributes to heart disease". There has been no credible evidence presented this is true. In fact more people are reported, by heart surgeons, to die with LOW cholesterol than high. Industry is unlikely to backtrack on their claim while vast fortunes are being made from Statins. In fact, the threshold for cholesterol was lowered, to scoop up millions more customers and place them on these drugs.

Dr Batmanghalidj, who wrote the book **'The Body's Many Cries for Water'** had this to say about the high cholesterol theory...

*'It is surprising that none of the frequently quoted and media-popularized doctors has reflected on the fact that cholesterol levels are measured from blood taken from the veins, yet **nowhere in medical literature is there a single case of cholesterol having caused obstruction of the veins.** Venous blood moves far slower than arterial blood and thus would be more inclined to have cholesterol deposits if the assumption of "bad cholesterol" were accurate. This mistake by us in the medical community, and its capitalization by the pharmaceutical industry, has caused an on-going fraud against society.'*

What about ADHD? They used to call children lazy, bored or mischievous. Now they are stamped with a psychiatric disorder. 6 million children are doped with Ritalin, in the U.S. This is disease-mongering and drug-peddling of the worst order. There is no attempt to reduce children's junk food intake and provide them with proper nutrition. No attempt to correct behaviour using good, old-fashioned discipline, either by parents or schools. No consideration given to the school environment which forces energetic youngsters to sit in fluorescent-lit holding pens and learn useless algebra. No actual evidence of a brain disorder. No attempt to remove 'excito-toxins' like sugars, glutamates, colours and flavourings from children's diet.

Parents and teachers accept the practice because a white coat has magical powers. *"No problem"*, the psychiatric sorcerers tell society. *"Give your kids this chemical cosh"* and *"Hey Presto!"* they are sedated. Don't they know the damage they are causing to the brains of these children? Why aren't parents up in arms over this? Polar Bears are shown more compassion.

In 1994 '**Gus**' the **Central Park Zoo** polar bear was seen obsessively swimming back and forth, for 12 hours a day, and was placed on Prozac. An animal behavioural therapist determined Gus was bored. The zoo redesigned his habitat to be more interesting and Gus' swimming obsession tapered off.

Like politics, a week is a long time in medicine and we all too quickly forget scandals, scares and empty promises. A serious dent in public confidence came about with the 'Flu' pandemic, otherwise known as '**The Great Swine Flu Caper**'. It might have succeeded in its goal of mass vaccinations across the globe, if not for the efforts of independent commentators on the internet exposing what they saw as 'a conspiracy by vaccine manufacturers to increase sales'. A German Magazine called the swine flu 'a total sham'. On the 3rd May 2106, The **British Medical Journal** reported…

'Key scientists advising the World Health Organization on planning for an influenza pandemic had done paid work for pharmaceutical firms that stood to gain from the guidance they were preparing. These conflicts of interest have never been publicly disclosed by the WHO'.

The WHO fuelled the fearmongering by stating 7 million could die. National governments purchased billions of dollars' worth of vaccines, which were never used. I was pleasantly surprised by the public's resistance. Despite a massive PR and marketing effort to get the untested Tamiflu shot, the public weren't convinced. After similar scares: SARS, Bird Flu, Swine Flu and the West Nile Virus (in each, the end of the world was nigh) there was a limit to which the public could be persuaded to roll up their sleeves.

The 2015 Ebola scare and 2016 Zika scare are simply iterations of the same push to shift product. The shenanigans of the vaccine industry raise a question. If the 'Swine Flu' pandemic was a fraud... and many believe it was... what other frauds have been, or are yet to be, perpetrated?

Trust is fundamental to the Doctor/Patient relationship. It is the principle reason patients allow doctors or surgeons to carve open chests, remove organs and mutilate breasts. Once trust has gone, the white coat will no longer have magical powers. Good doctors do not deserve to be tainted by the behaviour of corrupt colleagues.

"Medical science is the concentrated essence of Black Magic. Quackery is infinitely preferable to what passes for high medical skill."
- Mahatma Gandhi

Chapter 21
Crying Out For Change

The public is frustrated. I see it in the thousands of comments on health sites, blogs and social media. No longer are people prepared to unquestioningly accept. They are crying out for Doctors to:

Address cures, instead of managing symptoms.

Know the patient instead of relying on insignificant data points.

Be schooled in healing and prevention, instead of memorizing thousands of drug names.

Stop prescribing dangerous, marginally effective, or useless drugs, which require more drugs to manage the side effects of the first drugs, which trigger other conditions, requiring even more drugs... on and on... until we rattle when we walk and our vital organs give out, from toxicity.

Inform patients of the **true** risks of intervention.

Prescribe safer, less costly drugs.

Suggest alternatives with better prospects of healing.

Stop seeing us as a collection of independent parts, requiring separate medical specialties.

End over-medicalization, disease-mongering, unnecessary tests and bogus treatments, encouraged by bought 'thought-leaders', manipulated studies and junk science.

Stop drug companies 'inducing' Doctors to push their products. That so many Doctors accept inducements (bribes) is a scandal.

End the persecution of genuine healers by a vicious medical monopoly.

Provide truth and clarity in medicine. There is so much confusion people no longer know how to care for themselves.

End the patent system, which excludes natural compounds.

Demand alphabet agencies, like the FDA, CDC and AMA, serve the public, instead of being 'cesspools of corruption' and pharma industry 'gatekeepers', shutting out competition.

Alternative practitioners need to **stop** offering fad treatments, useless supplements and bogus 'Miracle Cures!'

Chapter 22
Health Freedom

There is something wrong, don't you think, when people are forced to travel to other countries, at great expense, to cure their disorders? The Mexican Cancer clinics come to mind. Having been to India, Thailand and other countries and seen, studied and experienced safe, natural treatments, I was amazed by the greater health freedom these countries enjoy.

In India, Ayurveda is government approved, as is Homeopathy and Gandhi's 'Nature Cure'. Hundreds of thousands of traditional healers, produced by the ancient 'guru' system, operate freely. 400,000 modern Ayurvedic Doctors are trained in both Western and Eastern Medicine. 20 years ago, the natural treatments I received in India were not available in the UK. Some of them are still not. Thank goodness for the internet. For all its faults, without it, we may have never heard of these safer alternatives.

Even with my knowledge and determination, it is difficult to find a skilled practitioner in the West and almost impossible to find one that will take on high risk patients. Some courageous healers operate under the radar but run the risk of prosecution for 'practicing medicine without a license'.

People should have the right to choose the health-care treatments and providers they desire. I imagine my mother, alive today, with Rheumatoid Arthritis. In a wheelchair, in constant pain. The Doctors can do nothing for her except pain management, using stronger and stronger drugs, with serious side effects. She cannot afford to travel abroad, as I did, for alternatives, even if she knew they existed (which she didn't). Her prospects are grim and she is going to die from the treatment (as happened). Now here I am, with two decades of knowledge of natural healing methods. I know what programs can heal her, safely, her symptoms would be gone, in as little as ten days. I have seen it on numerous occasions. Terrific. I can put my mother on the same program. Or can I?

According to my understanding of the law, if I help my mother, I am 'practicing medicine without a licence'. Even if she did all the actual work and I limited my contribution to nutritional advice, it could still be argued I prescribed 'drugs' to her. How so? Lemons, Turmeric, Ginger, Garlic, Chilli, Vinegar, Cabbage, Celery, Beetroot, etc., are 'food'. As long as these common items go into your salad, curry, or Spaghetti Bolognese, they remain 'food'. As soon as you use them for healing they transform, magically, into 'drugs' and drugs are the fiefdom of the **Food & Drug Administration** *(the enforcement arm of the pharmaceutical companies)*. Thus, a fundamental human right, exercised for thousands of years, is criminalized.

In 2005 the FDA warned cherry growers in the U.S. to stop making health claims about cherries. The cherry industry had received funding from the **Dept. of Agriculture** to do just that, in order to increase sales. The FDA was not amused. The cherry growers decided to fight and the **U.S. Supreme Court** ruled in their favour, admonishing the FDA. Not that this matters. If I felt I could save my mother, I would.

Vaccines

If you are one of those angry types, ready to toss squishy tomatoes at those you disagree with, better skip this section. No amount of evidence I present will reach you if anger or fear have shut down your critical thinking. I have put this under '**Health Freedom**', for reasons which should be obvious.

Time for a scary headline...

THEY ARE COMING FOR YOU!!

Do you have **any** idea what is coming down the line? The fight, by parents of vaccine-damaged children, to wake you up, is NOT just about protecting other children from damage. It is about the push for mandatory vaccines by the 'Big Pharma' gangsters and the politicians in their pockets. It is the push by these criminals to not only OWN your children's bodies. But yours, too. With **$Trillions** of dollars up for grabs, you can bet the farm mandatory vaccination WILL become law and it isn't going to stop at children. ADULTS are next.

Please tell me you get it? YOU will be required to 'catch-up' on all the shots you missed. There are around 250 MORE vaccines in development. Profits are stupendous with no downside for corporations. Is the rush to cash-in any surprise? They KNOW the public is going to resist, which is why we are seeing coercion already, with hospital workers forced to get useless flu shots or lose their jobs.

Authority-figures on TV keep telling you vaccines are *'safe and effective'*. This meme, like so many other memes, has been driven home, for decades. To the point it is now an article of faith. But faith is not science. It is religion. Like believing in the Tooth Fairy or Santa Claus or the Easter Bunny. You have never investigated what you are being told because you trust them. You trust them because you don't see the people who really run the industry. You see sweet nurses and smiley Doctors and vaccine leaflets that say the worst you can expect is a mild fever or a sore arm. This isn't science. It is MARKETING.

Complete strangers are injecting known poisons into your infant. When a child is damaged, as too many are, there is no apology, no compensation. YOU have to deal with the consequences, for LIFE. Not the sweet nurse. Not the smiley Doctor. Not those who inflict disease. You. Do you have ANY idea how devastating it is to raise a child with severe autism? Don't you think it is worth taking a little time out from Game of Thrones or some celebrity pap, checking to make sure it won't happen to you, or your child? Even if the risk is minor. A good place to start is,

'How to Raise a Healthy Child in Spite of Your Doctor' - *Robert Mendelssohn, MD*

Numerous vaccines are needed (it is claimed) to provide us with 'protection', when previous generations were robust enough not to require them. In the U.S., the total is now an outrageous 74 doses (53 injections) by age 17, an increase of 24x since 1950. Other countries don't vaccinate to this degree and some don't vaccinate infants, at all, under the age of 2. So why do we, when the U.S. has the worst infant mortality of all industrialized nations?

In 1989 TWENTY-SIX more vaccines appeared on the CDC schedule. In 1986, vaccine manufacturers became immune to ALL financial liability from the destruction of lives their vaccines caused.

It is **unnatural** to bypass natural defences, with poisons, which lodge and accumulate in immature brains and vital organs. Destroying neurons, displacing vital minerals, upsetting the 'microbiome', lowering IQ, creating 'excito-toxicity', Parkinson's, Alzheimer's, ADHD and a host of other maladies.

Are Vaccines Safe?

In 2011, when giving pharma corporations freedom from prosecution, for the damage their shots were causing, the **U.S. Supreme Court** pronounced vaccines, **'unavoidably unsafe'**.

The alarming rise in chronic disease, in our children, coincides with the increase in the vaccine schedule. Most of the diseases occurring are **listed on vaccine inserts** *(the inserts you and your Doctor never get to see)*. One vaccine insert has **42 paragraphs** of precautions and adverse reactions. Only **significant** reactions have to be listed. The Eli Lilly

Material Safety Data Sheet (MSDS) for Thimerosal states exposure to mercury, in pregnancy and in children, can cause:

"mild to severe mental retardation and mild to severe gross motor impairment."

Sounds very much like autism. DPT Vaccine maker, **Sanofi Pasteur Inc.**, includes the following in their package insert:

*"Adverse events reported during post-approval use of Tripedia vaccine include idiopathic thrombocytopenic purpura, **SIDS**, anaphylactic reaction, cellulitis, **AUTISM**, convulsion/grand mal convulsion, encephalopathy, hypotonia, neuropathy, somnolence and apnea.*

Autism and SIDS *(remember 'cot death' and 'shaken baby syndrome'?)* How many mothers were jailed for 'murdering' their babies?

Are Vaccines Effective?

If vaccines are effective, and the number of vaccines has increased dramatically, **why has the health of our children fallen off a cliff?** Mississippi has the highest rate of vaccination in the U.S. 99.4 percent. You would think Mississippi would have the healthiest population. Wrong. It has the WORST. Between 2012 and 2014 the state ranked **LAST** in overall health rankings.

We have all heard how diseases during the early part of the 20th century were eradicated due to vaccines... polio, smallpox, diphtheria, whooping cough, measles and tetanus. Yet those diseases were most gone PRIOR to the introduction of vaccination. Vaccines claim credit, when improved sanitation, better nutrition and health and safety at work were largely responsible.

I am old enough to remember, during childhood, none of my classmates had chronic disease. I never heard of cancer, diabetes, fibromyalgia, autism or auto-immune disease. Chronic disease affected older people. Sickness was limited to chickenpox, measles and mumps, which were considered mildly harmful. There was no such thing as ADD or ADHD. There were no psychological disorders. I only received 3 vaccines. Even so, I ended up with allergies, chronic anxiety and was painfully shy. Since then, Cancer has exploded from 1 in 1000 to 1 in 2. Autism from 1 in 5000 to 1 in 28.

Autism tends to get the most headlines. What is notable about autism is its remarkable resemblance to a disorder that plagued Europe, Australia and North America in the 50's, called **Acrodynia**. More commonly called '**Pink Disease**'. The cause of Pink Disease? Mercury. Medicines containing mercury were declared 'safe' and dispensed to infants when teething. 30% who were sensitive to mercury, died. Many more were irreparably damaged. How many of you have heard of Pink Disease? It was missing from my school books. How long did it take the authorities to identify and withdraw the mercury? Decades. How many cases of Pink Disease occurred after it was withdrawn? ZERO.

Another example of mercury in medicine is Calomel.

*'Medical uses for Calomel were common well into the nineteenth century. It acts as a purgative and kills bacteria (and also causes irreversible damage to their human hosts). Some treatments are of historical interest. The three physicians attending Gen. Washington's final hours administered calomel to the dying President. Lewis and Clark carried it on their expedition and used it to treat their men's STD's. Louisa May Alcott (author of Little Women) suffered from its effects. Even in the present decade several cases of mercury poisoning have been attributed to facial cremes containing calomel. Such cremes are banned in the United States because mercury is readily absorbed through the skin.'- **Loyola University, Chicago***

In 2003, after a 3 year study called '**Mercury in Medicine**', an investigative committee, chaired by U.S. Senator Dan Burton, filed its report. I won't go into all its findings, of which there are many, but I present one important correlation. Forget Dr Andrew Wakefield, the poster boy for establishment attacks (who will eventually be seen as a hero). **Symptoms of Autism match symptoms of mercury poisoning**.

Other alarming comments,

*'In July 2000, it was estimated 8,000 children a day were being exposed to mercury **in excess of Federal guidelines** through mandatory vaccines.'*

A lead researcher, regarding mercury being used as a preservative in vaccines, said this:

*"There are other compounds that could be used as preservatives. And everything we know about childhood susceptibility, neurotoxicity of mercury at the fetus and infant level, points out we should not have these fetuses and infants exposed to mercury. **There's no need of it in the vaccines.**"*

Let's not forget the views of parents, which the media are ignoring. If your child is normal before a vaccine and handicapped after, and nothing else changed, it can be reasonably assumed the vaccine caused the handicap. A bit like waking up to find snow on the ground. You didn't see it snow, there is no scientific study proving it snowed overnight. But there it is. Snow on the ground.

The maximum recommended level of mercury in water is 2 parts per million. Yet, the amount of mercury in vaccines was 51,000 parts per million. After 'realizing' the amount of mercury (Thimerosal) in the childhood vaccination schedule, recommended by the CDC, far exceeded all safety limits, the **American Academy of Pediatrics (AAP)** and the **United States Public Health Service** called for the immediate removal of Thimerosal from vaccines, on July 7, 1999.

In 2002 Members of Congress inserted a "hidden provision" into the **Homeland Security Bill** to prevent any lawsuits over Thimerosal. The **NY Times** reported:

'The Bush administration asked a federal claims court today to seal documents relating to hundreds of claims that a mercury-based preservative in vaccines, Thimerosal, has caused autism and other neurological disorders in children.'

And yet, at the height of the 2009 H1N1 flu pandemic, the medical industry called for pregnant mothers and infants to be injected with Tamiflu, which contained thimerosal. A 2014 report by a panel of eminent scientists concluded **Tamiflu was no more effective than paracetamol.**

At what point do we stop seeing negligence, or incompetence, and start seeing something more sinister?

NO amount of mercury is safe. Manufacturers have not removed mercury from all vaccines, 15 years after being asked to.

Why? Because, as happened with Calomel, these diseases would abruptly stop, leaving no doubt vaccines were the cause. In Denmark, thimerosal was removed from vaccines in 1992. **Autism rates decreased by 30%** as a result. *(I don't recall a word from the media).*

To hide the cause it becomes imperative to keep mercury in the system. How are they doing it? Via flu and hepatitis B shots. How 'safe and effective' are they?

*"There is no evidence that any influenza vaccine, thus far developed, is effective in preventing or mitigating any attack of influenza. The producers of these vaccines know that they are worthless, but they go on selling them anyway." – **FDA former Chief Vaccine Control Officer Dr. J. Anthony Morris.***

Hepatitis B is primarily a blood-transmitted disease, associated with unprotected sex with multiple partners & intravenous drug use involving sharing needles. Last time I checked, newborns weren't shooting up with heroin, at orgies. This is not a childhood disease.

After three years of Congressional Hearings on vaccines the **Subcommittee on Human Rights and Wellness of the Committee on Government** concludes:

"Thimerosal used as a preservative in vaccines is likely related to the autism epidemic. This epidemic in all probability may have been prevented or curtailed had the FDA not been asleep at the switch regarding the lack of safety data regarding injected Thimerosal and the sharp rise of infant exposure to this known neurotoxin. Our public health agencies' failure to act is indicative of institutional malfeasance for self-protection and misplaced protectionism of the pharmaceutical industry."

A growing body of evidence has found connections between high rates of autism and mercury in vaccines. **Scientific Papers Linking Thimerosal Exposure to Autism (10)**

Scientific Review of Vaccine Safety Datalink Information June 7-8, 2000, Simpsonwood Retreat Center, Norcross, Georgia

"···we have found statistically significant relationships between the exposure and outcomes" [...]

At 2 months - *an unspecified developmental delay.*

At 3 months - *Tics.*

At 6 months - *attention deficit disorder.*

At 1, 3 and 6 months - *language and speech delays.*

At 1, 3 and 6 months of age - *the entire category of neuro-developmental delays, which includes all of these plus a number of other disorders."*- **Dr. Verstraeten**

*"This association leads me to favor a recommendation that **infants up to two years old not be immunized with Thimerosal containing vaccines** if suitable alternative preparations are available."*- **Dr. Johnson**

*"The number of dose related relationships are linear and statistically significant. You can play with this all you want. They are linear. **They are statistically significant.**"*- **Dr. Weil, AAP**

In another revelation, CDC whistle-blower, Senior Scientist, **Dr. William Thompson,** *'openly admitted to taking part in altering scientific data at the CDC (Centers for Disease Control) to hide statistical links between vaccines and autism'.*

Apparently a large bin was placed in the middle of the room and relevant documents tossed into it. A documentary about it called '**Vaxxed**' was pulled from a New York Film Festival.

You can watch beheadings live on TV, all kinds of sadism and blood-letting but be shown information on vaccines? Sponsor of '**Vaxxed**', actor Robert de Niro, who has an autistic son, has called for the truth about vaccines and autism to be publicly investigated. The documentary '**Trace Amounts**' also sheds light on this issue.

Should We Get Vaccinated?

I cannot tell you what to do. Some of you, no matter what you read, will vaccinate, out of fear. You have been badly frightened by Hollywood and the media. Yet, what is it we fear? All these scares have us hiding under our beds, terrified of viruses flying around you never hear of again and which turn out to be less dangerous than the vaccines given to 'protect' us. Notice how quickly a vaccine is released after a scare? How does that happen, unless it is scripted? My own choice would be NO. Because, after looking into it, I believe vaccines do not protect against disease but induce it. You are supposed to make an INFORMED choice. How is that possible? We know industry buries negative findings and studies. How much confidence can you have in those telling you to get your shots, when they are all sucking on the vaccine industry tit? Like the Academy of Pediatrics or 'independent' spokespeople, like Dr Paul Offit, who infamously said babies can tolerate *"10,000 vaccines at once."* This is the man who will snaffle an estimated $46 million from the sale of a vaccine he was involved in approving. Apparently, he is now known as Dr Paul Proffit. ([20])

Every Doctor knows vaccines inflict disease. Parents TELL them. **Françoise Berthoud, MD**, a French paediatrician, studied rates of disease amongst vaccinated and unvaccinated populations of several countries and wrote a book about it called '**The Marvellous Health of Unvaccinated Children**'.

'Some of the basis of my ability to speak on the marvellous health of unvaccinated children comes from my personal experience as a medical doctor, having collected years of feedback.

"My child began coughing immediately after the vaccination."

"He has had constant ear aches since he was vaccinated."

"My 16 years old daughter is completely unvaccinated. She is almost never sick. If she does get sick, it's two days at the most."

"The neighbour's kids followed normal vaccination guidelines. They are constantly sick and on antibiotics."

'The Lesson Learned On Vaccination' (<u>11</u>)

"As a concerned, compassionate and considerate paediatrician, I can only arrive at one conclusion. Unvaccinated children have by far the best chance of enjoying marvellous health. Any vaccination at all works to cripple the chances of this end."

'The medical monopoly or medical trust, euphemistically called the American Medical Association, is not merely the meanest monopoly ever organized, but the most arrogant, dangerous and despotic organization which ever managed a free people in this or any other age. Any and all methods of healing the sick by means of safe, simple and natural remedies are sure to be assailed and denounced by the arrogant leaders of the AMA doctors' trust as fakes, frauds and humbugs. Every practitioner of the healing art who does not ally himself with the medical trust is denounced as a 'dangerous quack' and impostor by the predatory trust doctors. Every sanatorium who attempts to restore the sick to a state of health by natural means without resort to the knife or poisonous drugs, disease imparting serums, deadly toxins or vaccines, is at once pounced upon by these medical tyrants and fanatics, bitterly denounced, vilified and persecuted to the fullest extent.'
- J.W Hodge, M.D.

Chapter 23
Big Pharma

I was shocked, recently, when glancing at the list of side effects of a well-known skin ointment. One in particular stood out.

DEATH.

From using a skin cream?!

Welcome to the world of Big Pharma. A group of gigantic pharmaceutical corporations that, since their inception, according to **Peter Gotzsche**, medical researcher and head of the **Nordic Cochrane Center**, meet the criteria of organized crime according to U.S. law.

More than 70 percent of new drugs approved within the past 30 years originated from trees, sea creatures and other organisms. Some of them are things like draculin (an evocative name!) found in the saliva of vampire bats, and a hormone found in the saliva of the gila monster, a venomous lizard. While most are completely safe in their natural form, they are less so in synthetic form.

To remind you. At least 350,000 people die, per year, in the U.S. and Europe, from pharmaceutical drugs. There have been nearly 2 billion adverse drug reactions, while some drugs create additional disorders, such as diabetes. There is no doubt some are helpful but many are toxic. We know this. That's why we keep them out of the reach of children.

Millions content themselves with the relief pharmaceutical drugs provide. I've been immensely grateful for it, at times. Especially when it comes to pain. Relief makes bothersome symptoms go away. However, think about what this actually means.

Switching off the body's pain signal is like disabling a fire alarm going off in a building. The noise of the alarm is irritating, so we isolate the power and silence it. Later, another alarm may be triggered. We silence it again. Then, enjoying the silence, we sit back as the building burns to the ground. In the same way, we suppress symptoms, allowing disease to progress.

If I were the CEO of a drug company, mandated by law to make a profit and exempt from any liability if people are harmed, would I be disappointed, or pleased, if my vaccine caused millions of cases of asthma, allergies and autism? Or my fluoride-laced 'anti-depressants' triggered impotence and diabetes? Or radiation and chemo caused MORE cancer? If my 'blockbuster' drug suppressed one symptom yet triggered two more? Would I ensure these drugs are safe? Or would I stay quiet, rake in billions in profits and just pay the fines? ([12])

Judge for yourself...

'The European Commission has imposed record fines of 855.22 million euros (£534m; $753m) on eight pharmaceutical companies for operating secret market sharing and price fixing cartels in the supply of vitamins throughout the 1990s.'

The heaviest penalty of 462 million euros was handed out to the Swiss based multinational Hoffman-La Roche. The investigators maintain that the company was the chief instigator and was involved in all 12 cartels they uncovered.

Other mischief from the pharmaceutical companies...

- **GlaxoSmithKline** (2012): Illegal promotion of drugs. Fined: $3 billion (largest fraud fine ever).
- **Pfizer** (2009): Off-label promotion of COX-2 drugs including Bextra, Geodon, Lyrica and Zyvox, with *"the intent to defraud or mislead"* cost the pharma giant a loss of 90 percent of its 2008 income. Fined: $2.3 billion (then the largest fine of its kind).
- **Eli Lilly** (2009): The maker of Zyprexa has had several court appearances over the anti-psychotic drug, which Lilly attempted to attract elderly populations suffering from dementia to try. The sales team were directed to disregard the law. Several lawsuits in various states resulted. Fined: $1.4 billion, $25 million, and $22.5 million (reduced from $2 billion for violating use of a product label approved by the FDA).
- **Abbott** (2012): Abbott had no science to back up its target of the drug Depakote—an anticonvulsant—for use in treating elderly populations suffering from aggression and agitation related to dementia. But that did not stop the company from sending its sales reps into nursing homes. The company was also fined for promoting it as a treatment for schizophrenia although no scientific evidence existed to support that claim. Fined: $1.5 billion.
- **Merck** (2011): The painkiller Vioxx was eventually pulled from the market in 2004 for its connection with an increased risk of heart attacks. But before then, Merck illegally promoted it as a treatment for rheumatoid arthritis despite any official approval. The company also reportedly made misleading statements about Vioxx's effect on heart health. Fined: $950 million.
- **Allergan** (2010): Botox—the cosmetic toxin injected into the face to smooth out wrinkles and plump up lips—was misbranded by Allergan

as a treatment for pain, headaches and cerebral palsy. The ruling also found that the company paid doctors $1,500 to attend presentations on the drug's other uses in order to help the company push out its product. Fined: $600 million.

• **AstraZeneca** (2010): After misleading doctors and patients over the safety of its antipsychotic drug, Seroquel, which included known risks of gaining weight and developing diabetes. The company continued to deny any wrongdoing. Fined: $520 million.

• **Novartis** (2010): Between 2000 and 2001, Novartis used misbranded promotion of the drug Trileptal for treatment of neuropathic pain and bipolar disorder despite no approval for treating those conditions. Other Novartis drugs were also misbranded, including Diovan, Exforge, Tekturna, Zelnorm and Sandostatin. Fined: $422.5 million.

• **GlaxoSmithKline** (2009): Between 1997 and 2004, the company was investigated for off-label promotion of Wellbutrin SR, an anti-depressant that had been illegally prescribed for cases of bipolar disorder as a result of the company's marketing efforts. Fined: $400 million.

Fines a deterrent?

'Despite the large amount, $3 billion represents only a portion of what Glaxo made on the drugs. Avandia, for example, racked up $10.4 billion in sales, Paxil brought in $11.6 billion, and Wellbutrin sales were $5.9 billion during the years covered by the settlement, according to IMS Health, a data group that consults for drugmakers.' - **Dr. Peter Breggin**

Fancy a trip to Disneyland, Doc?

"GSK's sales force bribed physicians to prescribe GSK products using every imaginable form of high priced entertainment, from Hawaiian vacations to paying doctors millions of dollars to go on speaking tours to a European pheasant hunt to tickets to Madonna concerts, and this is just to name a few," - **Carmin M. Ortiz, U.S. attorney, Massachusetts.**

Wondering where your Diabetes came from?

Johnson & Johnson (2012) to pay more than $1.2 billion in fines. Prosecutors accused Johnson & Johnson and Janssen of hiding the risks associated with Risperdal, which is approved to treat schizophrenia, bipolar disorder and behavior problems in teenagers and children with autism. Side effects can include weight gain, an increased risk of diabetes and, in older patients, an increased risk of stroke.

The **New York Times** and **Huffington Post** had this to say:

'Although it is encouraging to see the legal system to some degree catching up with drug company malfeasance, there are a number of problems with the criminal and civil cases brought by the Department of Justice against drug companies. As in the case of the recent settlements with GSK, the company makes so much money from the drugs they are little affected by paying out even $3 billion. Its stock rose significantly after the announcement. Individuals within the companies, including the CEOs, rarely have to face individual charges or fines. None of the money goes to the victims of the civil and criminal offenses, including the many children injured by the fraudulent off-label marketing of drugs like Risperdal and Paxil.'

On 25th Feb 2016, British newspaper, the **Daily Mail**, carried this story… **'How Big Pharma greed is killing tens of thousands around the world'**.

The article contained a number of damaging charges:

- Too often patients are given useless - and sometimes harmful - drugs they do not need.
- Drugs companies are developing medicines they can profit from, rather than those likely to be the most beneficial.
- Commercial conflicts of interest are contributing to an *'epidemic of misinformed doctors and misinformed patients in the UK and beyond'*
- The NHS is 'over-treating' its patients. The side effects of too much medicine is leading to countless deaths
- The full trial data on statins – cholesterol-lowering drugs prescribed to millions – **has never been published**
- One in three hospital admissions among the over-75s is a result of an adverse drug reaction

The medical director of **NHS England**, Sir Bruce Keogh, admitted 1 in 7 NHS treatments – including operations – are unnecessary and should not have been carried out on patients.

Former editor of the **New England Journal of Medicine**, Dr Marcia Angell, revealed that of the 667 new drugs approved by the FDA between 2000 and 2007, only 11 per cent were considered innovative or improvements on existing medications. Three quarters were essentially copies of old ones

There is nothing new about their behaviour.

"New drugs present greater hazards as well as greater potential benefits than ever before—for they are widely used, they are often very

potent, and they are promoted by aggressive sales campaigns that may tend to overstate their merits and fail to indicate the risks involved in their use. . . There is no way of measuring the needless suffering, the money innocently squandered, and the protraction of illnesses resulting from the use of such ineffective drugs." – **Robert Kennedy, 1962**

There is much which could be written about 'Big Pharma' and its long-standing collusion with politicians, consumer protection agencies and media *('Print anything negative and we will withdraw our advertising dollars').*

"Drugs never have cured one single person having a disease of any nature. When it is asserted they have done so, it will be found on closer examination and argument that the person has recovered comparative health in spite of drugs and not through their influence."
- Kiki Sidwa, N.D.

Chapter 24
Why Alternative Medicine Fails

My bookshelf is stuffed with 'How To' books. **How to Cure Arthritis. How To Cure Cancer, Heal Your Inner Child, Scarf Tying Magic** (*don't ask me where THAT came from!*) I can't tell you the number of different therapies I tried over the years that did little to improve my condition. I was a sucker for every therapy out there. Cranial Osteopathy, Reflexology, Re-birthing, Reiki, Acupuncture, Past-life regression, biofeedback, Alexander technique, aromatherapy, homeopathy, hypnotherapy and supplements galore.

Finding a cure should have been easy. Instead, I became hopelessly confused. The more I learned, the more my mental bucket overflowed, the less able I was to make a decision. It wasn't until I encountered Ayurveda and Nature Cure that the clouds parted and I realized why all the alternative therapies had failed.

Imagine having a healing toolbox, where each tool is a different therapy. There is the **Nutrition** tool, the **Exercise** tool, **Emotional Healing** tool, **Stress Reduction** tool, **Herbal Supplement** tool and so on. There are a tremendous number of tools and therapists. Most therapies are really just small slices of larger healing systems. They rarely cure on their own because you need more than one slice. You need the whole system.

Allow me an illustration. You have a chronic disorder like diabetes, cancer, arthritis, cardiovascular or auto-immune disease. The Doctor can only manage, not cure it, so you decide to try alternatives. You have a session or two of acupuncture, reiki or aromatherapy, fix yourself a colourful salad, purchase the latest fad supplement, invest in a juicer, and start bouncing in the garden, trying not to land, head-first, into the ornamental fish pond. Nothing works. Why? It's easy to blame a therapy or therapist but the most common reason for failure is because you are practicing **Water Pistol Medicine**. What do I mean?

Imagine your house is on fire. You call the Fire Department in a panic. Minutes later you are relieved to hear the sound of a siren, only to look on in disbelief as a single fireman leaps out of the truck, holding a water pistol. Your house burns down.

Let's change the scenario. You call the Fire Department. The fire truck arrives. This time, teams of firemen attack the fire, from all sides, with multiple hoses, aggressively and continuously. They save the house.

Now, apply this scenario to your disorder. You attack your disease 'fire' with multiple 'hoses'… cellular and regenerative detox, massage, sauna, herbs, hydrotherapy, emotional and psychological healing, exercise, acupuncture, or other 'energy' medicine. You flood your body with nutrients, resolve toxic relationships, pay off debts, escape back to nature, de-stress and relax. With all these 'hoses', would you extinguish your disease 'fire'? You bet. You may not be able to afford all the different therapies, have time to apply them, or know exactly which to have in your healing toolbox, but at least you now know why you haven't been getting anywhere.

You cannot extinguish a raging inferno with a water pistol.

So, what CAN we do? Well, just as there is a fire brigade for fires, there is a fire brigade for disease. Detox, wellness or healing retreats. Nature Cure centres, ashrams, even spiritual retreats. Places which specialize in putting out disease fires. They can look at a fire, know how many hoses are needed and add more, as necessary. This is what we do with our '**30 Days to Health**' program, you will read about later. It uses many 'hoses'.

Another reason alternatives fail is what I call, '**Grasshopper Medicine**'. Due to financial constraints, or a lack of understanding, we try a therapy. It does not work, so we move to the next… and the next… and the next. We are like grasshoppers, hopping from leaf to leaf.

Yet another illustration… Imagine you are drilling for oil. You believe there is oil underground, so you sink a well. Then another and another and another. Unfortunately, you do not drill deep enough and never strike oil.

This is key. Not only do you need the RIGHT tools for the job, you need to give them a chance to work.

Why Supplements Don't Work

"Miracle Goji Berries!!

"Incredible Noni Juice!"

"Co-Enzyme Q10!"

"The Vitamin D3 Cure!"

Are you tired of supplements that don't work? Have you fallen for slick marketing?

We all have. There are thousands of chemicals and nutrients, in nature, for Health Marketeers to select from. Once they finish with individual nutrients, they can move on to combinations. The sky is the limit. Apple cider vinegar and baking soda, cinnamon and honey, turmeric and ginger. The public hand over money, convinced this is the solution they need. The supplements industry rakes in $BILLIONS.

In a sense we are blessed. Thanks to legislation that protects the industry, we have an embarrassment of riches whereby consumers can purchase virtually any herbal supplement they desire *(except those that cure cancer)*, without the intervention of a qualified medical practitioner or pharmacist. We are free to 'self-medicate'. "Bravo!" But there is a catch *(isn't there always)*. This blessing may be a curse. Over the years, there has been an explosion of over the counter products (OTC) available to the consumer. You can find thousands of suppliers of this and that herb, with prices ranging from reasonable to outrageous. This is part and parcel of living in a capitalist system. Retailers constantly vie for your attention. Last year it was Vitamin D. Today, Cherry Juice. Tomorrow, B17. Backed up with unlikely healing claims. The market is huge, profits spectacular, results pathetic.

What is the use of having thousands of different suppliers of Echinacea (an immune booster), when as much as 90% of Echinacea products have no Echinacea in them at all. Try it. Echinacea causes the tip of your tongue to tingle. Does this happen with the Echinacea you purchased from the health store?

In a Press Release in February 2015, the **New York Attorney General's Office** asked **Wal-Mart**, **Walgreens**, **Target** and **GNC** to halt sales of certain herbal supplements. 79% of their herbal supplements were found to have no herbal DNA. The worst offender was Wal-Mart, with 96% of their supplements having no DNA, from plants listed on their labels. Additionally, there were unlisted contaminants, not printed on the label. Rice, beans, wheat, house plants. That wonderful healing herb you are excited about? A dead house plant.

The leading brand of vitamins in the U.S. is called Centrum. Laboratory analysis recently found Centrum vitamins contain GMO, food dyes and toxic chemicals. Most High Street 'vitamins' are synthetic, inorganic and not the whole vitamin. Because there are no set standards for multivitamins, it would not come as a surprise if someone DID sicken or die from taking them. Children's versions are more hazardous.

When the media report on 'deadly' vitamins, you can be reasonably confident they are talking about **synthetic** vitamins, not natural. **Whole, natural vitamins do not cause harm.**

According to research by **Food Safety News**, up to 80% of honey sold in supermarkets and pharmacies has no trace of pollen. The small packages provided by restaurants and airlines have even less – 100%. The lack of pollen is due to ultra-filtering. Natural honey is heated intensely, filtered, then watered down, rendering it useless.

How many of you have purchased OTC herbs and supplements and seen a difference in how you feel? Medicinal herbs, in your typical health section, are often formulated with little, or no, therapeutic agent in the product. If, by chance you improve, it has nothing to do with what is in the product but the power of your own belief. The 'Placebo Effect'. It is curious how, when a farmer makes healthy claims about cherries, the U.S. FDA goes after them, all guns blazing but when food giants strip away all that is health-promoting and nutritious in our food, drench it with known carcinogens, there is not a word.

Were you aware some herbs can trigger a healing crisis? The medical term for this is 'Herxheimer Reaction'. When your immune system is sufficiently strengthened by a herb, it starts to 'clean house', releasing toxins into circulation. This may cause you to feel a little unwell. A healing crisis is actually a sign your vitality is returning... something to celebrate. Not knowing this, you mistakenly believe the herb or supplement is making you sick.

Opportunist lawyers, sniffing million-dollar awards, used healing crises to slap lawsuits on manufacturers, accusing them of harming patients. Manufacturers, due to the risk of litigation, were forced to dilute their products to the point where they no longer trigger a healing reaction, rendering them ineffective.

What other reasons might there be why an herb or 'Miracle Cure' won't work?

1. **Availability**. Herbs, from other countries, are blocked by Customs, to protect domestic markets. They might actually work!
2. The herbs may have no active oils present, due to oxidation. Or their healing properties have been destroyed by processing.
3. There may not be any herb in the product.
4. Supplements companies have replaced 'live', organic, natural ingredients with 'dead', synthetic chemicals and crushed rocks. These are cheaper to manufacture and do not degrade. They also do nothing for you.
5. The recommended dose isn't sufficient to bring about the intended outcome. One person may weigh 120 lbs and require 2 tablets 2x daily, while another may weigh 240 lbs and require double that.
6. You are comparing herbal supplements to pharmaceuticals. When you don't experience a rapid enough response, you quit. Herbal remedies can take longer to work than pharmaceuticals.

Were you aware of this? I certainly wasn't.

There is one factor, not yet mentioned. Perhaps, the most important. You.

I once encountered an overweight, middle-aged man, in a road-side café, tucking into a plate of sausage, egg, bacon and fried bread, washed down with a cold beer. I noticed the pills next to his plate. *"For my heart"*, he said, flashing me a beaming smile. Once finished, he lit up a satisfying cigarette. I was shocked this man would believe drugs could protect him at the same time he was eating artery-clogging food, drinking and smoking. As if one negates the other. It does, I suppose. The food, alcohol and cigarettes were negating any benefit from the drugs.

This is the appeal of Health Industry marketing. *'Do not worry. Continue your disease-inducing lifestyle. Just take our pills.'* A message sending you straight to the morgue.

If you are smoking, drinking too much alcohol, eating poor quality food and not exercising, why would you believe taking a pill, herb, or supplement, will undo all that harm?

Making Herbal Tinctures

Herbs work. Thousands of years of trial and error have shown us. Modern medicine is founded on herbal medicine. But where to find high quality herbal supplements? You could seek out an herbalist, who will formulate a remedy, tailored specifically for you. If you are the enterprising type, make your own. The quality will be outstanding. The best outcomes occur when using wild-crafted herbs, prepared locally, picked at the right time and taken in the right dose. Search online for how to make your own herbal remedies. Herbalists don't want you to know how easy it is!

At 6 am, during a full moon, you might observe me gathering bunches of a Thai herb called 'Luk Tai Bai' (Phyllanthus Amarus). 30 minutes after being picked, half of the herb will be bottled in grain alcohol and the remainder, already drying, will be made into a tea. In those 30 minutes I will have stripped all the leaves and placed them in a blender filled with 700 ml of 40% proof, grain alcohol. After blending for a few seconds, the mixture is decanted into a sealable jar. Kept out of direct sunlight, in 3 months it will be ready for use.

Why make your own herbal tinctures?

1. Tinctures are the most potent form of herbal remedy.
2. The quantity of herb used can be vastly more than commercial products. While they may use 10% herb and 90% alcohol. Mine are 60% herb and 40% alcohol.
3. Better quality. Fresh, organic, picked by hand. No old leaves, twigs, fillers, chemical residues or 'stabilizers'.
4. The potency will be vastly superior to commercial products, if you harvest when plant healing factors are at their peak (lunar gardening).
5. It costs very little. No customs charges or shipping costs. You get more for less!

Phyllanthus Amarus is one of the most useful herbs in the Thai herbal kingdom. Beneficial to the liver and kidneys, it is a wonderful daily tonic for diabetes and hypoglycaemia. It lowers high blood pressure, relieves stress, insomnia and anxiety, is excellent for blood detoxification, gallstones, prostate and pancreatic disorders. It is a tonic for the stomach and frequently prescribed for fevers and back pain. Powder from leaves, twigs or roots can be taken as a tea. Making herbal remedies is easy. Try it with your favourite herbs.

Poor Attitude

I have encountered numerous people, sceptical about alternative healing. These people have little tolerance for techniques such as EFT.

"Tap my head while I am talking? Hahaha!"

The dictionary definition of a cynic is:

'A person who believes people are motivated purely by self-interest rather than acting for honourable or unselfish reasons.'

A sceptic:

'A person inclined to question or doubt all accepted opinions.'

Cynicism and scepticism will absolutely block you from receiving the benefit of, what I have found to be, extraordinary tools. Yes. There are perfectly good reasons for not trying a particular technique. You may not feel comfortable with the practitioner. Or it may be too expensive. However, if your reasons are due to fear, ignorance or blind prejudice, you might wish to re-evaluate your beliefs.

Cynicism and/or scepticism kept me on damaging anti-depressants for years, closing me off to therapies, like EFT. If I had remained closed, I would never have healed.

Where are you in your thinking? Are you a sceptic or cynic? Ask if your thinking is helping or hindering you?

Destructive Humour

For 20 years, I was a military man, immersed in a culture of sarcasm and mocking humour. Men in uniform are merciless when making fun of each other and I was a Master of the art. Sarcasm and cutting humour were not confined to barracks. Wives and girlfriends were often on the receiving end. At home or in front of others. When Patti and I married, she had no idea what she was letting herself in for. Every time we met up with friends, she would be teased. She tried to take it in good spirits and be 'one of the lads' but eventually broke down, crying.

"You are destroying my self-esteem", she said.

"Don't be daft. We are just having fun", I responded.

After a few days of chewing it over, I realized she was right. This was a new world to her and military humour can be cruel. I decided I would no longer use my wife as the butt of my humour. Having taken this decision, I was able to stand back. To be an observer rather than participant. I began to notice the hurt in the eyes of wives and girlfriends of my friends, which caused me to see them in a new light. I lost respect for them. My wife had forced me to grow up.

Anyone knowing me would be surprised at this transformation. When you have been behaving in a manner which is normal, to you, you aren't really aware of any other way of being, so don't consider, or believe, it is possible to change. I owe Patti a big thank you. Because of her I became a better person.

From Cynicism to Love

Growing up with a hypochondriac mother and alcoholic father is going to have an effect on any young mind. In complete contrast to the compassion I show, today, I was as cold as ice when it came to anyone being ill. Years of observing my mother had drained me of sympathy. She would often faint in public, always falling toward me. Duodenal ulcer, hiatus hernia, heart problem, arthritis. Conversations constantly revolved around her health. Like all children, I wanted my mother to be normal. I resented the fact she wasn't, eventually cutting her out of my life completely.

Eight years after doing so, I was hit by a mid-life crisis. Unresolved feelings toward my mother were part of my unhappiness. So, I resolved to face her, armed with a list of complaints I wanted to rectify. When we met, my plan did not go well. It became clear my mother was not going to change. I was left with a difficult decision. Walk away and never come back, or find a way to accept her. Overcoming my frustration and disappointment, I acted with a maturity I had seldom shown before and made a vow to myself.

"No matter what my mother says, from this day forward, I am going to love her".

Mum lived two more years and died from real, not imaginary, disease. Had there not been a reunion, I would have been racked with guilt and remorse. Instead I found myself at peace. My mother had not changed. I had. Instead of fighting for the mother I wanted, I surrendered and accepted her, 'warts and all'. Surrender brought me forgiveness, tolerance and peace of mind. No longer was I emotionally cold when faced with those who were ill. The last two years of my life with my mother were a blessing.

There is a powerful lesson here. Very often we think anger, rage and the power of our will, will bring us what we want, when what is REALLY needed is for us to surrender. If you are unhappy, look for where the resistance is, in your mind. Then let it go.

Stewart's Bypass

Stewart was a Type II diabetic, with osteoarthritis in his hands. After 6 days of a 7-day detox, I saw Stewart, looking seaward, from the veranda, a puzzled expression on his face.

"That's odd. I can see more clearly without my glasses".

Stewart had done detoxes before but this was the first time his eyesight had improved. I put this down to the power of bitter herbs, particularly Bitter Gourd, which works wonders for diabetes.

"Great news", I said. *"Just keep taking bitter and reduce sweet."*

A couple of years later Stewart returned. His glasses firmly back on his nose. He had not altered his lifestyle. His diet was poor and there was major tension in his marriage. Furthermore, Stewart needed a triple-coronary bypass. Understandably fearful of going under the knife, I explained to him about the Dean Ornish Heart Program and how it successfully reversed heart disease, in under 18 months, using diet, exercise, stress reduction and group support and that, if he adopted it, he would be out of danger quickly. As Dr Ornish reports:

*'Comprehensive lifestyle changes cause a 91% reduction in angina and significant improvements in myocardial perfusion and ventricular function **after only 1 month.**'*

"Really? How come my Doctor never mentioned it to me?"

Good question. I suggested Stewart go with the Ornish protocol but add steps to speed up the process. Heart repair herbs; contrast bathing/hydrotherapy; sauna and massage; castor oil packs; fasting with fresh, raw juices. By doing this, 12 months might come down to 9… 6… 3… or even 30 days. Stewart liked the idea and opted for a 30-day program. Alas, he was extremely restless. After six days he left and flew to the UK, underwent the operation and spent the next year recuperating, counting his blessings he was still alive. Another heart patient, with him in intensive care, had died on the operating table. I met Stewart part-way through his recovery. He wasn't a happy man.

"I wish I had stuck with the program".

'Years from now, people looking back at us will find our acceptance of the HIV theory of AIDS as silly as we find the leaders who excommunicated Galileo.'
Kary Mullis, Nobel Laureate

Chapter 25
Useful Techniques

'Sudarshan Kriya' is an advanced yoga breathing exercise. One description says about it,

'This unique breathing technique eliminates stress, fatigue and negative emotions such as anger, frustration and depression, leaving you calm yet energized, focused yet relaxed.'

Benefits like this sounded great. I was keen to give Sudarshan Kriya a go. Little did I know what I was letting myself in for. The exercise is practiced for 10 minutes, each day, as part of the **Art of Living** program. However, what excited me was the extended session, lasting 30 minutes, which is particularly powerful.

How does it work? After a few loosening stretches, you sit on a chair in a darkened, quiet room and breathe in and out, in a controlled, rhythmic fashion. A few slow breaths to start. Increase to medium pace. Then fast.

Slow, Medium, Fast.
Slow, Medium, Fast.
Repeat for 30 minutes.

It is quite a workout. For the first 25 minutes I noticed little difference in how I was feeling, beyond the exertion. Then, during the last few minutes, as my lungs were working hard, I could feel the tips of my fingers and toes beginning to tingle and my body flooding with 'Prana'. Prana is the 'life force', or 'energetic' aspect of air, the Chinese call 'Chi' or 'Qi'. It is taken in through the breath and circulates to all cells. The tingling sensation moved up my limbs, until my whole body felt energised. It is difficult to describe. I had never experienced anything quite like it.

The 30-minute session completed, I lay down on my back, in the Yoga 'Corpse Pose', as instructed, keeping absolutely still, eyes closed. A light blanket was put over me. All was quiet. After a few minutes, someone in the group started giggling and then one by one we followed suit until everyone was cackling like hyenas. Laughter is infectious!

The first three times I completed this exercise nothing really happened for me. On the fourth occasion, I decided to go for broke and put maximum effort into the breathing. The additional effort paid off. By the time I lay down, I felt super-charged with 'prana', my whole body tingling and vibrating like a tuning-fork. After 10 minutes of lying completely still, mind lost somewhere in 'space', I heard a low moan emanating from within the room. The hairs on the back of my neck stood up. This was altogether different to cackling hyenas. The fearful moan increased in intensity, until it turned into a scream. I suddenly realized the person who was screaming was me.

What had caused me such terror? At the point my moan intensified into a scream, I became aware of a dark shape, just above my upper chest, moving slowly toward my feet. The fear was intense as the shape exited my toes. Then, suddenly, it was gone. The room was quiet as I looked at the others in self-conscious embarrassment. I must have seriously spooked them. I asked the leaders of the group what happened.

"We do not try to interpret", came the unsatisfactory reply.

Whatever had been weighing so heavily on me was gone. I felt light on my feet and in my spirits. Dissatisfied with the answer (thinkers **need** to know) I determined to find out what it was. An answer came from a Sufi priest I met, two years later, on one of my jaunts abroad (Sufism is the mystical aspect of Islam).

"It was a Jinni", he declared.

Have you seen Aladdin and his Magic Lamp? Aladdin rubs the lamp and out pops a Genie. According to Arabic mythology, a Genie or 'Jinni' is a supernatural creature that can be good, bad or neutral. Akin to 'demons' in the Bible. Not a very nice thought learning my slim carcass had been occupied by a malevolent being. I wondered when and how such an entity could have entered me and then recalled an incident, four years previously. It was at the time I was 'in the pit'. That dark place, filled with despair, suicide and hopelessness, when my nervous system was completely 'burnt-out'. I had woken up from a fitful sleep and sensed a shape at the foot of the bed. Just as happened during the 'Sudarshan Kriya' exercise, the hairs on the back of my neck stood up. I remember watching, in frozen alarm, as a dark, indistinct shape entered my body, through my feet, moved up my legs, until it stopped at my chest. I shrugged the incident off and went back to sleep, telling myself it was just a nightmare. But was it? During nightmares people wake up before the plane crashes, they are about to be murdered, or fall out of the sky when flying. Not this time. I was awake when the 'possession' took place.

What had this 'Jinnie' been up to for four years? Perhaps ensuring I stayed 'in the pit'. I did wonder when I went through my Christian conversion, whether the voice I heard, screaming at me not to go through with it, had been the 'Jinnie'.

I rarely tell the story of this DIY exorcism, for obvious reasons. Western minds have been trained to dismiss such things. They are scornful and dismissive. Asians, on the other hand, who love ghouls and ghosts, have no difficulty believing at all.

After this experience, my opinion of Christian retreats, revivals and spiritual workshops, changed. Previously, when my wife and I had attended evangelical revivals, we would observe people falling down, writhing on the floor, giggling or shrieking. At the time I thought they were all completely barmy. I still think some of them are. However, I am far less sceptical today than I once was.

Remarkable, unique, intense, rhythmic. Sudarshan Kriya was an amazing, 'supernatural', eye-opening experience.

It is fair to say Sudarshan Kriya addresses the **Spiritual Layer**.

EFT + NLP

EFT (Emotional Freedom Technique) is a very simple method for dissolving emotional issues and curing addictions. Using the tips of your fingers, you tap on certain energy meridians, in a specific sequence, while focussing on the trauma, addiction, or fear, you wish to dissolve. EFT has been described as 'acupuncture without the needles'.

NLP (Neuro-Linguistic Programming) is a way of providing shortcuts to success in life by altering our thinking and beliefs. To look at what thoughts hold us back and what thoughts advance us. The word 'programming' sounds a bit creepy but it is not that at all. Therapists identify the negative language we use and encourage us to replace it with positive statements.

How do the two work together? If I am scared of spiders and say to my conscious mind, *"I am NOT scared of spiders"*, it does not work because my subconscious mind has *"I AM scared of spiders"* written to its internal hard drive. I am now 'in two minds', which only creates internal conflict. This is where EFT and NLP work together beautifully. EFT, for reasons I have yet to understand, but do not really care, as long as it works, dissolves the emotion attached to a belief, reducing its power to the point a new belief can be inserted. In other words, delete 'I am scared of spiders', using EFT, then insert 'spiders don't bother me', using NLP.

In my experience, EFT+NLP has a 70% success rate. Way in excess of anything Psychiatry achieves and without the need for medication. It costs very little and results can be had within minutes.

The Power of Miracles

'MIRACLE CURES!' Don't you just love them? Available online, for a one-time-only bargain price, guaranteed to cure every ailment.

'Snake Oil' salesmen draw us in with fantastical claims and testimonials, of this and that miracle cures, selling DVDs, books and products. They might have worked for the seller but they do not work for us. We are not all the same.

The King of Miracles was Jesus. If we could only touch the hem of his garment, we would all be healed. As a child I was an angelic choirboy. Later, like the Prodigal Son, I lost interest in the Church. It seemed archaic and out of touch and the media (including Hollywood and the music industry) have done a good job of destroying religion. Singers, like Madonna, Beyonce and Lady Ga Ga, are 'Satan's little helpers'. These Baphomet Belles, crucifixes around their necks, dress like sluts, and shriek, while pumping their hips and grabbing their crotches, spellbinding millions of impressionable pre-teens. In the UK only about 4% of the population remain regular Churchgoers. You know the Anglican Church is lost, when missionaries start coming to the UK from Africa.

How did the four great world religions get to be as popular and powerful as they are? Despite all the negative stories we hear, which are less to do with religion and more the corrupt leaders within it. Maybe, just maybe, they know something we do not. Is it possible Miracle Cures do exist? There are plenty of examples in health. Every 'incurable' disease cured. Every 'spontaneous remission' is, if you think about it, a miracle.

My family knows something about miracles. Especially my daughter, Lauren.

The Last Rites

In 1990, Lauren was born, seven weeks premature, in a British Military Hospital, in Hong Kong. She was 3lb 4oz. The fact she was born at all was itself a miracle. A Naval surgeon in Hong Kong (I was based there at the time) had conducted a D&C (scraped the womb) of her mother, when 8 weeks pregnant. How he missed a 1" foetus we will never know. My wife knew she was pregnant, she had our son, Michael, previously. Two over-the-counter pregnancy tests were positive. Unfortunately, the hospital's pregnancy test was negative, so that was that. They would not listen and went ahead with the procedure. My wife was devastated, believing she had lost our child. What relief we felt when my wife's uterus continued to swell. Although followed weeks of worry, wondering if the foetus had been damaged. A later complaint, by us, led to the hospital updating their tests.

Lauren was duly delivered, fingers and toes intact. Within days of her birth, she contracted double pneumonia. Her lungs became so stiff the incubator in the Special Care Baby Unit could not inflate them. She had to be hand-ventilated by nurses, round the clock. At one point her lungs burst, like balloons, with the pressure. One morning, around 4am, the hospital called us.

"Sorry. Please come quickly! She will not last the hour".

In dread, we rushed to the hospital, arriving just before the final moments. Our daughter lay, grey and lifeless, her major organs failing. The Doctors had made every effort to save her, even injecting adrenaline directly into her heart. I looked at them. They shook their heads. The end was close. A kindly priest had rushed to administer the last rites. I was stunned. This could not be happening. Consumed with grief, I cried,

"God, please save her!"

The words came out as an unintelligible cry of anguish. Then something happened no-one has been able to explain.

Lauren's heart-rate picked up, then grew stronger.

She survived.

Crab Fishing

Four years later, I flew our children to America to visit the theme parks. Disneyland, SeaWorld, Universal Studios and so on. At one point in the holiday we drove to Washington State to visit my wife's hermit-like father who lived, in a small log cabin, on the edge of a lake. A charming man, he showed the children how to catch crabs by attaching chicken legs to a hook, then casting them into the lake, from the jetty. They loved it, as most children would. I was sat up at the house, watching, when Lauren called out:

"Daddy! Daddy! Watch me catch a crab!"

Lauren cast into the water and, to my horror, still holding the rod, followed the chicken into the lake, disappearing under the surface. I raced down from the house, watching to see if she came up but she didn't. I dived in and desperately felt around, water too murky to see anything. Dread enveloped me. So many children drown in these lakes. My searching became desperate. I came up for air then plunged down again. At this point, even if I did find her, would she still be alive? It felt like an eternity passed as I frantically groped for her.

"I can't find her. I can't find her. Please, God. PLEASE God. Help me! HELP me!"

Then, suddenly, I felt a strand of hair, grabbed more, then knew I had her. Thrusting as hard as I could, we surfaced.

Watching my daughter's lungs empty of water, then breathe, was an indescribable relief. Later my son and I tried to make light of the incident by buying her a crab pendant with moving claws.

It is perhaps fanciful of me to wonder if she still has it.

Peace of Mind

I still pinch myself at what happened that night, in a quiet, country English Abbey. For a decade I had suffered chronic anxiety, panic disorder and depression, trying all kinds of therapies, with little progress. Then, in one night, like a puff of smoke, it was gone. Anxiety, panic, suicidal thinking, depression. All of it. Gone. Replaced by an indescribable peace of mind and sense of wellbeing.

How was this possible?

Like many people today, apart from Baptism and a Church wedding, my relationship with the Christian Church was non-existent. Feeling the strain of our daughter's struggle for life, I had started making tentative steps toward the Church. For the next 4 years, I was like a fish on a hook, slowly being reeled in. Why did it take so long? I needed to meet people who spoke and acted normally. Not speaking medieval language, driven by Messianic zeal, to convert me.

Later, after re-marriage, I went from Church to Church, attending evangelical revivals, some of which were truly inspirational. Yet I couldn't bring myself to commit to what was on offer. Speaking in tongues, falling down on cue, singing 'happy-clappy' tunes in praise of a murderous Zion, raising hands high in the air, hugging strangers my instincts told me I should run away from. My chest was too tight, voice too monotone and personality too introvert to play singalong.

One day my wife and I were invited to a 'Marriage Review' weekend run by CARE, a charity which supports family life. A series of workshops had been arranged, to breathe life into stale and stuffy priests' ossified marriages. Our own marriage was in serious trouble, despite us providing pre-marriage counselling to love-struck youngsters with no clue what they were getting into. They were 'in love' and thought that was all you needed for marital success. John Lennon was wrong when he sang 'All You Need is Love'. Money is the number one cause of divorce.

The instructors for the course were refreshingly down-to-earth. One in particular impressed me. I explained my chronic stress problems to him and how I could not understand why I wasn't able to bounce back. He related his own experience of anxiety. Born in a prisoner-of-war camp, his parents had been executed by the Japanese. He presented a simple choice:

"It is up to you. You can spend eight years with a psychiatrist and get nowhere, or spend eight minutes with God and be transformed".

Hmm… This is what you call a 'no-brainer'. It was crunch time. Nothing ventured, nothing gained. After the workshop completed, we found an empty room, where this man led me through a brief, spoken ritual. I repeated his words:

"Father, I do not have the strength to do this alone, the burden is too heavy. From this point on I hand everything over to Jesus".

It was disappointing. No heavenly host of angels. No flashes of lightning. No transcendent experience… Jesus standing before me… with holes in his hands. I do recall something highly unusual, though. My mind was **screaming** at me, NOT to do it. I almost capitulated and walked out. Instead I did something I had never considered before. I told my mind to *"Shut up!"*

"Is that it?" I thought, and went to bed.

The next morning, I was not the same person.

I cannot recall a time, throughout my life, ever being at peace. My 'Monkey Mind' was always over-active, out of control. Buddha described the human mind as being filled with drunken monkeys, jumping around, screeching, chattering, carrying on, endlessly. In Asia they say 'foreigners think too much'. They are right. Westerners have given primacy to the mind, to logic, reason and science. I saw my restless mind as a curse of intelligence. Now, all the worries, chatter and negative thinking, so much a part of my life, were gone. Replaced by an incredible peace of mind and a feeling, as if floating on air.

I tried to rationalize what had happened. Handing your problems over to someone else will naturally lighten your burden. It is logical. Yet, this was something very different. A supernatural peace. What the Bible calls '**The Peace that Passeth all Understanding**'. It cannot be explained. You have to experience it.

American, Billy Graham, was a charismatic, Christian evangelist and spiritual adviser to several U.S. Presidents. Billy knew how to work a crowd. At large rallies, he would encourage people to come forward to be converted. More than 3 million did so, over the years. After one particular religious revival, those who had come forward were asked about their conversion experience. Most said the ecstatic state lasted about two months before evaporating. Those, whose transformations became permanent, had immersed themselves in Christian life. They became selfless instead of selfish, helped others, read the Bible, joined the Church, prayed, and gave thanks to God for their salvation. They did not do as I did and ride the feeling, thinking it would last forever.

Priests would tell me how blessed I was and to hang on to it. I did not understand what they meant. Once it was gone, I understood. It is the same phenomenon I experienced in retreats. When you remain in Church, ashram, healing retreat, detox centre, or gym, it is easy to stay on track. You have support from those around you, access to knowledge and the feeling of being part of a large family. However, once you leave, you become like a hot coal that spits out of a roaring fire. Away from the heat, it quickly goes cold. Isolated, you struggle to maintain the lifestyle changes. Your enthusiasm and interest fade.

I am sure that incredible peace would have lasted longer, had I stayed within a supportive environment (this is why we provide follow-up support to our retreat guests). Instead I could not overcome the difficulties I had with organized religion. I felt closer to 'God', sat under a tree, than on a Church pew. The conflicts in my 'rebound' marriage had not resolved and my career in Information Technology came with 'Expect burn-out' in the Job Description.

All these things and more chipped away at my 'supernatural' peace, until it was gone, never to return.

My 'miraculous' transformation had lasted nine months.

Chapter 26
Do You Want to Be Cured?

What a question. Everyone wants to be cured. No they don't. I can see the ones who are ready to die. Note the resignation in their faces. They have lived their lives, had their careers, seen their children grow up and leave home. They feel too old, too sick, too tired, or too depressed, to summon the energy to fight. An end to sickness would be a relief. Death holds no fear.

Some believe they don't **deserve** to live, convinced illness is retribution for some past misdeed. Death or suffering the price they must pay for mistakes in life. Convinced by authority-figures their disorder is incurable.

Then there are those who gain financially (from the State) or emotionally from being sick. They have been ill for so long they do not know who they would be without their disease. In a wheelchair, or on crutches, they receive attention and sympathy. Without it they are part of the anonymous crowd. It is difficult to shed disease that gives you benefit. A part of you will sabotage your efforts.

Have a good look at yourself and ask whether you truly wish to heal? Because if, deep down, you don't, it is better not to waste the time of others, better spent helping those who do. I see this with alcoholics. They come to see me, adamant they want to stop drinking. From experience, I have learned 9 out of 10 cannot be helped. Alcohol has a vice-like grip on them. They need to reach rock-bottom before the message, *"you are killing yourself and destroying the lives of your loved ones"*, sinks in. Only then can they be helped.

I can no longer do it. It is too painful to put heart and soul into helping drinkers, only to see them self-destruct. Organizations like Alcoholics Anonymous (AA) are better able to assist.

Chapter 27
The Power of Belief

You have probably heard of the '**Placebo Effect**'. This is where the power of your belief heals you. The Doctor gives you some sugar pills, tells you it is "medicine" and you get well. The 'Placebo effect' is accepted by the Medical profession even though not fully understood.

When it comes to the power of positive thinking or 'mind over matter' Doctors tend to describe the idea as 'New Age twaddle,' or the latest scornful label, 'woo'. This is how their minds have been trained. 'Doctor Brain'. This is curious when there are numerous **officially recorded** incidents of patients being healed from 'incurable' diseases. Doctors call them 'Spontaneous Remissions'. There is a database for them, although when you investigate, there is nothing 'spontaneous' about them at all. Individuals play a full part in their cure.

The **Spontaneous Remission Project** has been put together by the **Institute of Noetic Sciences** and has over 3500 case studies published in the medical literature of people who experienced spontaneous remissions from seemingly 'incurable diseases.' Most of the case studies involved Stage 4 cancers where conventional treatment was declined or patients were given treatment, deemed by doctors to be inadequate for cure. There are also case studies of those who recovered from other 'incurable' diseases, such as heart failure, autoimmune disease and HIV.

Dr Lissa Rankin, an American physician who has investigated self-healing, has this on her website...

'Dr. Lissa Rankin was a skeptical physician, trained in evidence-based academic medicine and raised by a closed-minded physician father. But after witnessing patients who declined conventional medical treatment, only to experience spontaneous remissions from seemingly "incurable" illnesses, she couldn't deny the possibility that patients might hold within them the power to heal themselves. Her curiosity led her to dig deep into the medical literature to scientifically prove that the mind can heal the body. Her search uncovered not only proof that you can heal yourself, but also the shocking physiological mechanisms of how emotions like fear, loneliness, pessimism, and depression can make the body sick, while love, intimate connection, optimism, and faith can cure you'.

Dr Rankin reports approximately 30% of patients, given placebo, will heal 'spontaneously'. This, of course, is fantastic news because it confirms positive thinking should be part of any healing protocol.

Take care, though. The 'Placebo Effect' has an evil alter ego. The **'Nocebo Effect'**.

What happens when someone is given a Cancer or AIDS diagnosis? They already start to die. I have met people like this. A friend has advanced Emphysema and is convinced he is going to die. You can the resignation in his eyes. Education changed his mind but he took a lot of convincing.

Dr Rankin has other cases where patients, informed of the side effects of a drug, have gone on to manifest those very same side effects, even though they had been given sugar pills. Could this be the real reason Doctors rarely tell you of drug risks? Unlikely but it would be nice to think so. This is important.

BELIEVING you will sicken, or die, can **CAUSE** you to sicken or die. **BELIEVING** you are well and will live, can **CAUSE** you to become well and live.

Watch what you believe.

Chapter 28
Forget the Apple. I Want Relief!

No matter **how** much we are begged or cajoled, we refuse, or simply cannot change our ways. NO fruitarian detox. NO raw vegan diet. NO juicer. NO '30 Days to Health' Program. NO exercise. Forget it.

I wrote this book for those who were serious about healing and prepared to do whatever it takes to get well. Yet, I know, unless you have the support you need, only a small % of people will manage to change their lifestyle. The majority will NOT adopt a raw vegan diet, juice-fast, go on a Whole Food, Plant-Based (WFPB), Ketogenic, or even Paleo Diet. Fair enough. While I may be tempted to ease you out the door and leave you with your disease, **I hate to see such a large % of you suffer unnecessarily**. So, instead of writing you off, let's try and bring a little cheer.

If you recall, I am suspicious of isolated supplements marketed as 'cure-alls'. Noni juice, Acai berries, Spirulina, extract from the gall bladder of a Tasmanian Devil. Isolates can create even more imbalance. Yet, there ARE substances, virtually unheard of in alternative healing, with impressive records of reversing a wide spectrum of chronic diseases. Before I explain what they are and why they are impressive, I would like to present another view of sickness.

Imagine your body is a bucket, filling up, over the years, perhaps decades, with toxic sludge. You know the list by now... chemicals, heavy metals, metabolic wastes, inorganic minerals, undigested protein particles and acids. Eventually the bucket starts to spill over and we experience symptoms of chronic disease. Due to the poor state of our 'inner soil' (toxic, acidic, deficient, congested) our bucket becomes home to worms, flukes, amoeba, bacteria, viruses, mycoplasma and fungi. These freeloaders of nature, besides causing infection, inflammation and blocking nerve and lymph channels, produce their own waste, adding to our **'Total Toxic Load'** (TTL).

What would happen if, instead of major lifestyle changes, to create the perfect 'inner terrain', we cleared all this toxicity, or **TTL**, to the point symptoms disappear? We haven't altered what made us sick, so expect some disorders to return, further down the road. However, we obtain relief and often a cure because our body's 'septic tank' (the lymphatic system) is no longer so clogged and backed up. Our bucket has been emptied. Unlike U.S. President, Donald Trump, we have managed to 'drain the swamp'.

To reduce our TTL, there are three steps. Addressing any one of them will bring improvement. Addressing all three can work wonders.

1. Eliminate parasites… worms, flukes, viruses and fungi.

2. Remove toxic chemicals and heavy metals… mercury, lead, aluminium, fluoride, bromides, chlorides, plastics, excess sulphurs, glyphosate and glutamates.

3. Clear out the physical blockages and sticky accumulations (undigested proteins) Ayurveda calls 'Ama'.

Would doing these 3 things really resolve our health problems? According to a great number of past and present personal testimonies, the answer is an emphatic "Yes". *(It seems logical it would.)*

Have you realized yet I am talking symptom-relief? What I complain allopathic medicine does. However, instead of medical Weapons of Mass Destruction, such as fluoride, sulphur, mercury and aluminium-laced pharmaceuticals, we use anti-parasitic, anti-fungal solvents, at low doses, which can penetrate and soften those sticky and hardened deposits and clear them out. What solvents? There are a few. On top of distilled, or Reverse Osmosis, water, I will mention just two:

Drum roll…

1. Borax

2. Turpentine

"Cockroach spray and paintbrush cleaner? You jest!!"

No, I do not jest.

You should know by now industry fearmongering has little to do with reality and is intended to keep us away from substances that might help us. I have tested turpentine and borax on myself and did just fine. No writhing on the ground in agony as my kidneys and liver dissolved. "The dose makes the poison" and the amounts we are talking about are too small to cause harm.

Borax

Nothing can be more frustrating than to eat right, exercise, do everything you are told is necessary to restore health, and get nowhere. Could it be the reason you fail to improve lies with a mineral deficiency? A trace mineral you have never heard of?

Boron is one of four magnificent minerals, the other three being iodine, selenium and magnesium, which belong in everyone's survival kit. Boron is one of the foundation blocks of the body. It helps activate, or cause, many other functions to happen (13). It acts like a taxi, helping deliver calcium and magnesium to their proper places.

Found mostly in bones, heart and parathyroid, boron is essential for bone metabolism and proper function of endocrine glands (i.e. ovaries, testes and adrenals). It is strongly alkaline with a pH between 9 and 10 (pH 7 is neutral). It is a naturally occurring mineral and the major ingredient of a laundry detergent called Borax. Borax has good antiseptic, antifungal and antiviral properties.

Due to poor diets, malabsorption, cooking, and overuse of fertilizers, boron deficiency is widespread, especially in the soil. In zero-boron Jamaica, arthritis rates are 70%... even the dogs are limping. In the U.S., where boron intake is only 1-2 mg per day, arthritis rates are 25%. In high-boron Israel, where intake is 10-30mg per day, arthritis rates are half of 1%.

Boron in our cells is easily displaced by aluminium, which we are being bombarded with, in food, water, cosmetics and vaccines.

For optimal health we need 60 minerals, 16 vitamins, 12 amino acids, and 3 essential fatty acids (omega 3 & 6). Deficiency does not just apply to boron. Many other nutrients are badly depleted or missing from the soil. If we wish to be well, it is important to ensure we are assimilating ALL nutrients.

Is Borax a 'Miracle Cure'? I could write a book of testimonials with the conditions it is credited as resolving. Here are some, customers reported, as **improved** or **resolved**, using Borax:

1. Breast, Cervical, Lung and Prostate Cancer
2. Diabetes (Most physicians aren't aware Boron plays a part in sugar metabolism)
3. Osteoarthritis, Rheumatoid Arthritis, Juvenile Arthritis, Psoriatic Arthritis and Lupus (Systemic Lupus Erythematosus)

4. Osteoporosis and weak or broken bones (think hip fractures)
5. Poor concentration, memory and "brain fog"
6. Wound healing (75% faster)
7. Depression, hay fever
8. Asthma
9. Signs of aging on the skin (Liver spots, wrinkles)
10. Worsened menopausal and PMS symptoms
11. Allergies
12. Weak muscles
13. Stomach and digestive parasites
14. Candida infection and yeast infections (leaky gut, vaginal thrush)
15. Eye infections and poor vision
16. Pain and inflammation
17. Low Testosterone (attention bodybuilders and aging Lotharios!)
18. Calcification of tissue, including the pineal gland (Borax binds to and eliminates fluoride)
19. Insomnia
20. Autoimmune Disease
21. Psoriasis and Eczema
22. Bloating and abdominal pain
23. Chronic Sinusitis
24. Restless legs, flashes, night sweats

Borax also works because it is alkalizing. Many health problems arise when the body is too acidic, such as fungal overgrowth. Borax is very effective against fungi.

"Ok. Ok. But what's the point of taking it if I am not going to change my ways and all my disorders are going to come back?"

Symptoms are unlikely to return if the original cause is Boron deficiency. Once your symptoms resolve, instead of stopping Borax completely, switch to a maintenance dose of 3-6mg per day. This will prevent deficiency diseases arising.

In the 1960's PhD Dr Rex Newnham developed arthritis. A plant scientist, Rex discovered boron deficiency in plants and started taking 30 mg of Borax a day. In three weeks all pain, swelling and stiffness disappeared. He was able to cure a 9-month old girl, with juvenile arthritis, in 2 weeks. Such was his success, after 5 years, with no advertising, he was selling 10,000 bottles of borax tablets per month.

When this was discovered by the pharma companies, Borax was declared a poison and banned.

Sample Testimonials

*"As an ex runner I was told **my knees were shot** and needed replacing. At the time I was working in Russia and a local pharmacist advised to try this before knee surgery. Mix one box of baking soda with an equal amount of Borax. Blend and use 1 teaspoon in a quart of green tea and drink the whole thing every day. I was on a 3 month rotation, 1 off 3 on. At the end of 3 months my knees felt fine. I went home and had both x-rayed. Bone had returned to normal, cartilage was no longer stretched like an old rubber band and most importantly my Synovial fluid had gone from gone/gone to normal. In Russia Borax is widely used."* – **A. Jackson, North Dakota**

*"Amazing. I'm 51 and for 25+ years I had **severe psoriatic and osteoarthritis** and various related/resulting conditions like **hay fever, depression, anxiety, addiction, eczema, tinnitus** … Three and a half months ago, I started daily with 4 teaspoons of borax solution (one teaspoon of borax mixed with a liter of water) and 500 mg of magnesium (for the first ten days I took 1000 mg of magnesium). (Since I thought I also might have Pyroluria, I included zinc, B6, D3 and an Omega 6 supplement.) All my conditions are at least 90% better. The herx'ing was tiring at times, especially in the third month when it was most severe."* – **BoraxBeliever of Shorewood, WI, USA**

*"I was experiencing a horrible **auto immune condition** called **HS (Hidradenitis Supperativa)**. Very, very painful and debilitating. I decided to try the borax protocol to attack the autoimmune condition. In six weeks all symptoms of my condition had disappeared and it is 10 months later and I continue to be healed."* – **Kristina, Arizona**

Another forum contributor suffered with **Fibromyalgia/Rosacea, chronic fatigue and TMJ** for over 10 years which she believed was caused by fluoride. She used 1/8 tsp of borax and 1/8 tsp of sea salt in a litre of de-chlorinated water, and drank this for 5 days each week. Within two weeks her face cleared, the redness faded, body temperature normalized, energy level increased, and she steadily lost excess weight. The only side-effect was an initial aggravation of her Rosacea symptoms.

*"7 years ago **thyroid cancer**, the next year **adrenal fatigue**, then **early menopause**, the following year **uterine prolapse** followed by*

*hysterectomy – the following year **fibromyalgia and neuropathy**. Early childhood was fluorinated water along with fluoride tablets. Fall of 2008 I was looking at **total disability**. I could barely walk and couldn't sleep because of the pain and was throwing up daily from the pain in my back. After reading about fluoride I came to understand where all of my problems originated. I began the borax detox of 1/8 tsp in a litre of water and within 3 days my symptoms were almost gone."*

Walter Last has numerous reports of success (14) ranging from cancelling surgery for hip replacement, to removing **brain fog**, and curing **autoimmune diseases**. One woman wrote of curing her **Lupus** and **serious kidney disease** in 4 months with half a teaspoon of daily borax powder.

Fungi and Fluoride

Being an excellent fungicide, it is not surprising borax is successful in treating Candida. Walter informs us:

*'In normal healthy conditions Candida exists as harmless oval yeast cells. When challenged, chains of elongated cells called pseudohyphae develop, and finally strongly invasive long, narrow and tube-like filaments called hyphae. These damage the intestinal wall, and cause inflammation and Leaky Gut Syndrome. Pseudohyphae and hyphae can be seen in the blood of individuals with cancer and autoimmune diseases. Candida can also form tough layers of biofilm. This same study shows boric acid/borax inhibits the formation of biofilms and also the transformation of harmless yeast cells into invasive hyphal form. [...] I have shown **this process, commonly initiated by antibiotics, is a basic cause of most of our modern diseases**, and this makes borax and boric acid primary health remedies.'*

If, as some believe, fungal infection is a major cause of chronic diseases, like cancer, Borax is clearly a must-have weapon in your cancer-killing and prevention arsenal.

Borax, like Lugol's Iodine solution, can also be used to **remove fluoride and heavy metals from the body**. Fluoride not only causes bones to deteriorate, but the pineal gland to calcify and thyroid to become underactive. Borax reacts with fluoride ions to form boron fluorides which are then excreted in the urine.

In some countries Borax can still be found in the laundry and cleaning sections of supermarkets. There is no "food-grade" Borax available or necessary. According to reports, all commercial Borax is the same and "natural".

What and How Much to Use

As you will find, from testimonials, different dosages work for different conditions. As long as you do not exceed 1500mg daily, there should be no risk. My own preparation uses around 120mg per day for chronic disease.

Use as an essential Mineral: Firstly dissolve a lightly rounded teaspoonful (5-6 grams) of borax in 1 litre of good quality water. This is your concentrated solution keep it out of reach of small children.

Standard dose = 1 teaspoon (5 ml) of concentrate. This has 25 to 30 mg of borax and provides about 3 mg of boron. Take 1 dose per day mixed with drink or food. If that feels right then take a second dose with another meal. If there is no specific health problem or for maintenance you may continue indefinitely with 1 or 2 doses daily.

If you have a problem, such as arthritis, osteoporosis and related conditions, cramps or spasms, stiffness due to advancing years, menopause, and also to improve low sex hormone production, increase intake to 3 or more, spaced-out, standard doses, for several months, or longer, until you feel your problem has sufficiently improved. Then drop back to 1-2 doses per day.

For treating Candida, other fungi and mycoplasmas, or for **removing fluoride from the body** – using your bottle of concentrated solution:

Low dose for low body weight: 100 ml or 1/8 teaspoon of borax powder or 500 mg; best with or after main carbohydrate meal.

Medium dose for heavier individuals or more pervasive Candida: 200 ml or 1/4 teaspoon/1000 mg of borax powder; take with or after 2 meals.

High dose for strong fungal/Candida problems such as **autoimmune diseases, cancer or dementia**: ½ tsp of borax powder mixed with food.

Always start with a lower dose and increase gradually to the intended or effective maximum. Take the effective amount as long as required for 4 or 5 days a week, or interrupt for one week each month, or periodically alternate between borax and another fungicide.

Vaginal thrush: Fill a large size gelatine capsule with borax and insert it at bedtime for one to two weeks. Alternatively the powder can be mixed with cool solidified coconut oil as a bolus or suppository. With **toe fungus or athlete's foot** wet the feet and rub them with borax powder.

Walter Last says for boron to be fully effective in reversing tissue calcification, magnesium is required. For elderly individuals he recommends 400 to 600 mg of magnesium together with daily borax supplementation, spaced out during the day. With protracted joint problems additional trans-dermal magnesium. Oral magnesium may need to be adjusted according to its laxative effect.

You may take borax mixed with food or in drinks. It is rather alkaline and in higher concentrations has a soapy taste. You can mask this with lemon juice, vinegar or ascorbic acid. Drink the water spaced out during the day, for 4 or 5 days a week, as long as required. Ensure you are using either distilled, or Reverse Osmosis (RO) water.

My mixture is either 50/50 Borax + Baking Soda or a concentrated solution of Borax + Sea Salt + Vit C + Selenium + Iodine + Magnesium. For issues with scar tissue, cysts, plaquing of arteries and fibroids, I add Serrapeptase, a proteolytic enzyme, derived from the silkworm, which acts like a popular computer game 'Pacman', gobbling its way through dead, decaying and abnormal growths in the body, clearing obstructions.

Turpentine

'At the age of 31, an Austrian woman, Paula Ganner, with cancer metastases and colon paralysis after surgery, had been given two days to live by her doctors. She remembered that in Eastern Europe kerosene was used as a cure-all, and she started taking a tablespoonful each day. After three days, she could leave the bed, and 11 months later she gave birth to a healthy boy. At age three, this boy contracted polio which she cured with one teaspoon of kerosene daily for eight days. Ganner started spreading the information about the amazing results of using kerosene for all kinds of health problems, and over the years she received **20,000 thank-you letters with success stories.**'

20,000 success stories are certainly impressive. More so, when you consider the many who will not have written in. Here are some testimonials reported in the German magazine "7 TAGE" between September 1969 and February 1970:

*A dog had a **growth** the size of a child's fist on his neck and was given kerosene on sugar cubes. After two weeks, the growth disappeared.*

*After breast cancer surgery, a woman (48) developed **tumours in the uterus**. After taking a daily teaspoon of kerosene she could stop using morphine, and after six weeks she aborted three tumours.*

*Another woman took a teaspoonful of kerosene three times daily for two weeks, and repeated this after a two-week interruption. This not only cured her **stomach ulcer**, but also, to her surprise, her **diabetes**.*

*A man cured a **severe prostate problem** (it is not mentioned if it was cancer) by taking one teaspoonful of kerosene each morning and evening for four weeks. Later, he overcame a **stomach ulcer** in the same way. His son successfully used kerosene to cure a **chronic bladder problem**, and he cured his dog of **leukaemia** after a seven-week kerosene cure.*

*After a woman (60) had her right breast removed, **cancer** started in her left breast. She periodically took a teaspoonful of kerosene three times daily for two weeks and then paused for 10 days. She had no more cancer problems and no more fear of cancer.*

*A young woman (35) was sent home to die with an inoperable **large tumour in the pancreas** that extended to the adrenal glands. On the fourth day home, she briefly awoke from a coma and was given a* *spoonful of kerosene. Hours later she showed the first signs of improvement, and after four days she wanted to get out of bed. The kerosene cure was continued for another 10 days before she was investigated at the hospital in Graz and later discharged as being healthy.*

*After six days of using kerosene, a woman discharged dead tissue which was confirmed to consist of **dead tumour cells** (the type of cancer is not mentioned). After 14 days, the typical smell of terminal cancer disappeared. She took kerosene for 32, 25 and 14 days, with nine days of rest between each. As a pleasant side-effect, she was also cured of her **rheumatic problems**.*

*A woman (68) had **high blood pressure, heart and circulation problems and rheumatism**. She could hardly walk. After four weeks on kerosene, she was asked by a friend what she was doing to look suddenly so much younger. People think she is in her 40s. Her husband, who used to have a **bent back**, now runs like a youth. When she sometimes gets some pain in cold weather, she rubs her body with a sponge dipped in kerosene and lets it dry; this quickly removes any pain.*

*A woman with **colon cancer** was scheduled for colostomy (to remove her colon and have a bag fitted). Instead, she started taking teaspoons of kerosene. Not much was happening, so she took about 50 ml in one go, together with a lot of honey in milk. This was followed by four hours of diarrhoea with pus and blood and the abortion of her tumour.*

Other testimonials include overcoming **bone cancer, osteoporosis of the spinal column, severe digestive and gastro-intestinal problems, constant vomiting, rheumatism** and **sciatic problems**.

Until recently, I had never heard of kerosene or turpentine being used for health. Turpentine and kerosene have been used medicinally since ancient times. In Nigeria, 2/3rds of the population use turpentine as a 'cure-all'. In the 1800's the British and other navies carried kerosene, as a common medicine. In France, kerosene is known as *huile de Gabian* and is prescribed as a remedy for bronchitis, asthma and cystitis. Our own medical literature contains clinical studies by reputable researchers showing kerosene to be effective against cancer. The 1899 Merck Manual informs us turpentine is effective for a wide range of disorders including gonorrhoea, meningitis, arthritis, abdominal difficulties and lung disease. 100 years later, it says not a word about these cures. Only dire warnings regarding kidneys and lungs.

The reason kerosene and turpentine are successful is, in part, due to their effectiveness against microbes and fungi.

Most kerosene, today, is derived from petroleum, not wood, it is not recommended to be used medicinally, unless for an emergency and no other remedy is available.

How to Take Turpentine

The turpentine to use is '100% pure gum turpentine'. NOT the stuff you find in the hardware store.

1. Slowly pour a level teaspoon of turpentine over sugar cubes, or a rounded teaspoon of white sugar, to soak it all up. Then chew the cubes or soaked sugar and wash the mixture down with water. This clears the blood of pathogens.

2. Combine 1 tsp turpentine with 1 tsp castor oil, or another carrier oil, this will direct the turps into the GI tract and clear the bowel of pathogens. Normal gut flora are not harmed.

I like to use castor oil because it helps moves the bowels. It takes around 4 hours for the smell of turpentine to clear and any diarrhoea to stop. Plan accordingly, if you wish to go out.

Dr Jennifer Daniels discovered American slaves kept themselves free from disease, using turpentine. (20) Dr Daniels recommends following these steps twice a week for several weeks, but initially, daily, with long-term candida or chronic disease. Continue until the problem is fixed. She suggests preparing by drinking lots of water, adopting an anti-candida diet and cleaning the bowel. Ideally, while on the program, have three daily bowel movements but at least one.

Sources: **The Candida Cleanser** - Dr Jennifer Daniels. **Kerosene – A Universal Healer** - Walter Last.

An obvious question when considering Turpentine or Borax is whether you have parasites? Review the following list of common symptoms of infection.

If you believe you may have parasites, consult a health practitioner for further discussion and testing.

Do You Have Parasites?

1. Chronic fatigue for no apparent reason
2. Swollen or achy joints
3. Increased appetite, hungry after meals
4. Eat out at restaurants
5. Nervous or irritable
6. Restless sleep/teeth grinding while asleep
7. Night sweats
8. Blurry, unclear vision
9. Fevers of unknown origin
10. Frequent colds, flu, sore throats
11. Recurrent feeling of being unwell
12. Constipation
13. Diarrhoea alternating with constipation
14. Thinning or loss of hair
15. Allergies, food sensitivities
16. Irritable bowel, irregular bowel
17. Rectal, anal itching
18. Bloating or gas
19. Abdominal or liver pain/cramps
20. Mucus in nose that is moist or encrusted
21. Dark circles under the eyes
22. Bowel urgency
23. Skin problems, rashes, hives, itchy skin
24. Vertical wrinkles around mouth
25. Kiss pets, allow pets to lick your face
26. Go barefoot outside the home
27. Travel in 3rd world countries
28. Eat lightly cooked pork/ salmon products
29. Eat sushi, sashimi
30. Swim in creeks, rivers, lakes
31. History of parasitic infection
32. Loose stools or diarrhoea
33. Pale, anaemic or yellowish skin
34. Foul-smelling stools
35. Low back or kidney pain
36. Indigestion, malabsorption

Chapter 29
Cures

When a Doctor tells you, *"There is no cure"*, he is being honest. He just forgot part of the sentence...

*"**To my knowledge,** there is no cure"*.

Doctors are ignorant of alternative methods of healing. Their lack of knowledge is odd when healing systems like **Traditional Chinese Medicine** and **Ayurveda** have been healing for thousands of years. Are we really to believe the positive aspects of natural healing have already been incorporated into conventional medicine?

If I were to ask a natural healer if I can be cured, I would receive a very different answer:

"Of course".

Why the difference? The **Conventional Doctor** attacks symptoms, is lost without a diagnosis and never addresses underlying cause. He has already made up his mind what is wrong, within 2 minutes of seeing a patient. He isn't interested in knowing the patient.

The **Natural Healer** treats the **whole** person. Seeks to identify and resolve underlying cause and success does not depend on a diagnosis. He or she takes time to understand the patient.

How can the natural healer be so confident? Because they see clients, abandoned by conventional medicine, recover their health, time and again.

Note: Natural Healer is any practitioner bringing about healing without resorting to drugs or surgery.

Countless examples are to be found of those who have healed serious disorders. There are at least 350 known natural cancer cures. Hundreds of herbs and foods have proven anti-cancer activity. Research supports many of them. So does the historical record.

Renee Caisse and **Harold Hoxsey** cured tens of thousands of cancer patients, using Essiac Tea and the Hoxsey herbal formula, over several decades. Renee Caisse was seeing 300-500 patients a week, while Harry Hoxsey had 17 clinics and the support of the public, congressmen and even some Doctors. He eventually fell afoul of the high priests of medicine who refused to investigate his methods and hounded him for decades, despite two federal court judgments stating the treatments worked.

Dr Richard Schulze cured himself of serious heart disease, then thousands of the most severe cancer and chronic disease cases, before being raided and brutally shut down.

Dr Sebi was cured of asthma, diabetes, impotence and obesity, and then went on to heal many others.

Dr. Dean Ornish's Program for Reversing Heart Disease is the first program scientifically proven to reverse heart disease by making comprehensive lifestyle changes.

Dr Gabriel Cousens, at the Tree of Life centre in Arizona, has been curing Type II Diabetes, with raw food, for 30 years.

Arnold Ehret cured his disorders with fasting and fruit.

Dr William David Kelley healed his own cancer and thousands of others, through detoxification, diet and enzymes.

There are many others who have been successful in healing chronic disease. If we wish to heal, the Greats have shown us the way. A word of caution when researching these men. **Do not make idols of them.** Blind devotion or 'Guru-worship' and 'following the crowd' may not always produce the benefits we seek. In that case, travel a different path. There are many roads to Rome.

Dr Sebi

Dr. Sebi was born Alfredo Bowman, on November 26, 1933 in the village of Llanga in Spanish Honduras. He never attended school and came to the United States as a self-educated man, having been diagnosed with asthma, diabetes, impotence and obesity. He weighed 291lbs. After unsuccessful treatments with conventional doctors, Sebi was led to an herbalist in Mexico. Healed of all his ailments, Alfredo was inspired to also become an herbalist. Creating natural compounds, designed for cleansing and revitalization. of all cells making up the human body. His approach to healing with herbs was shaped by 30 years of practical experience. For Sebi, juice and water fasting were key. Dr Sebi fasted for 57 days. In 1988, a case against Sebi, for 'practicing medicine without a licence' was thrown out by the Supreme Court, after 70 witnesses swore Sebi's methods cured them of a wide range of disorders. Sebi believed mucus to be a major cause of disease. Mucus can harden and block the channels. Eliminate mucus-forming foods from your diet and you will heal. This idea is not new.

Arnold Ehret

100 years ago, Arnold Ehret wrote about his **Mucusless Diet Healing System**. Few people today have heard of Arnold, or his system. Arnold taught college until he was drafted for military service. After nine months he was released because of 'neurasthenic heart trouble'. He resumed his teaching career at 31, despite chronic ill health, suffering a kidney disorder and Tuberculosis (TB). Under the care of 24 different physicians at one time or another, Ehret eventually turned to natural methods, vegetarianism and mental healing but without completely satisfactory results. A stay in Nice, living on a milk-and-fruit diet, was only partially beneficial. The following winter, Ehret traveled to Algiers, living almost exclusively on the plentiful native fruits. His condition rapidly improved and he was emboldened to try short fasts, to aid the cleansing properties of the fruit and climate. Not only did Arnold regain his health but unbelievable energy, strength and joy of living. He and a companion undertook an 800-mile bicycle trip from Algiers to Tunis, returning completely exhilarated.

Dr Richard Schulze

'Dr. Schulze is one of the foremost authorities in the world on natural healing and herbal medicine. He holds a Doctorate in Herbology from the School of Natural Healing and a Doctorate in Natural Medicine. Dr. Schulze also holds a degree in Herbal Pharmacy and degrees in Iridology. He is certified in eight different styles of "body therapy" and has three black belts in the martial arts. Dr. Schulze has written numerous research papers on the topics of Botanical Pharmacognosy, Pharmacology and the making of herbal preparations.' At 11, Richard's father died in his arms, of a massive heart attack. At 14, his mother, the same. They were both 55. At 16, Richard was diagnosed with a genetic, 'incurable', heart deformity. Rather than accept the same fate as his parents, Richard worked hard on healing himself. Within 3 years, Richard had repaired his heart. Inspired to learn everything he could, Richard studied under the great healers. Dr. John Ray Christopher, America's greatest herbalist of the last century; Bernard Jensen; Paavo Airola and Dr. Kurt Donsbach, the renowned nutritionist. Richard took on thousands of patients, with the most serious diseases. His reputation grew until officialdom violently shut him down. In his book '**Common Sense Health and Healing'** Richard says,

"My clinics were open, spanning three decades, over 20 years, with over 20,000 patient visits in this country and abroad.

In the last decade of my clinical practice I specialized in degenerative and life-threatening diseases. Especially the ones medicine says are incurable, like cancer, AIDS, heart disease, arthritis, diabetes, liver and kidney failure, Alzheimer's disease and other neurological diseases. The news of my success with these patients and their life threatening diseases spread. My clinical success became an embarrassment to the medical community, and my patients thriving instead of dying became embarrassing living testimonials to the failure of modern medicine. I was arrested and my clinic was boarded up."

Richard's Wiki page was deleted by a conventional Doctor, for spurious reasons. There are countless examples like these, of famous healers, as well as testimonials from ordinary people, attending retreats and centres, with chronic illness who, failed by conventional medicine, healed themselves. Their stories inspire and give us hope. Richard Schulze's Incurable program includes a minimum of 12 days fasting. Richard believed 80% of people were healed just by properly cleansing the bowel. Other Doctors I have high regard for and you may wish to research, are Dr William David Kelley, Dr John Bergman and Dr Robert Morse.

Of all the successful healers I have researched, there is not one whose reputation, methods and successes have not been disparaged, diminished or dismissed. The charge of choice is that healing claims are not supported by scientific evidence. I hope I have shown this charge to be bogus.

The health industry wants us to believe cures are always 'just around the corner'. I wouldn't hold your breath. While there are encouraging signs some mainstream Doctors are opening up to alternative viewpoints, for a conservative health industry to suddenly become trailblazers and bring cures to us, is as unlikely as arsonists coming up with proposals to extinguish a blaze they started. It is not going to happen until money stops corrupting the system. Pressure for change has to come from the bottom-up. This pressure is set against entrenched and powerful vested interests whose profit models, control and very existence, depend on the maintenance and expansion of disease.

Medicine is a business, and cancer, the biggest business of all. 70 years and vast amounts of money and research since the 'War on Cancer' was launched and they still do not know what causes cancer (so they claim). They force the same deadly treatments on patients as decades ago and refuse to entertain, or investigate, alternatives. It is a strange system that crosses its fingers in the hope the cancer dies before the patient and in which shrinking a tumour is lauded as a 'success', even when the patient dies.

With little sign of help from mainstream medicine, the patient has to look elsewhere. Due to the monopoly power of the **Medical-Industrial-Complex**, solutions can be hard to find. We have to travel abroad, or fix ourselves.

That's ok. We can do it. We are in the **Bypass Age**.

7 Elements of a Healing Plan

Let's start with the basics. Recovering your health is like renovating a home. If you feel like a dilapidated building, with crumbling foundations, you are going to need some restoration.

1. **Good architectural design** (Your healing program)
2. **Materials** (Supplements, herbs, supportive therapies)
3. **Project Manager** to keep reconstruction on schedule, come rain or shine. (Health professional/friend/family member)
4. **Prepare the ground** (Cleanse and detoxify)
5. **Put in strong foundations** (Flood the body with nutrients)
6. **Build** the walls, put on the roof. Install plumbing, electrics and windows (The 5 Layers of Healing)
7. **Keep your home in good order**. (Healthy lifestyle, resolve minor problems before they become serious disorders)

For those who are highly stressed, easily discouraged or seeking instant fixes, this already seems like hard work. It is not. The only difficulty is having the confidence and motivation to get on with it.

Which Methods?

A little research will already have convinced you healing is possible. Which methods to choose? There are hundreds. I have selected four.

Remember reading 80% of disorders will resolve, simply by properly cleaning the bowel? Arguably, if you have cleared the body of waste and pathogens, you may already have done enough to resolve your disorder(s)..

1. **Water Cure**. As simple and affordable as you can get.
2. **Reversing Diabetes**. Equally simple. On our 'Reverse Diabetes' retreats, I see Type II Diabetes and pre-diabetes (hypoglycaemia, hyperglycemia and metabolic disorder) reverse within 7 days and 100% resolved, within 21 days, just by a change in nutrition.
3. **Auto-Urine Therapy**. This will surprise you.
4. **'30 Days to Health' program**. The core of the healing protocol I used to cure myself and which can be applied to just about every chronic and degenerative disorder that exists.

All four methods can be undertaken at home. The latter has the most steps. However, each step serves a purpose, is easy to understand

and apply. **If you are not seeing the results you expect**, you may be following the program correctly but are not being aggressive enough.

A well-designed holistic detox/cleanse is at the core of natural healing. In my experience, 10 days is the minimum needed to see results with chronic disorders and the minimum time required to kill off parasites and fungi, if fasting. Standard anti-Candida protocols will kill fungi (also known as thrush or yeast infection) but can take 3 months or more to work and the candida, too often, returns. It is quicker and more effective to try the solvents, or fast on juices (read Angela's story).

A parasite cleanse needs a little thought. People can be host to a variety of parasites including fungi, flukes, amoeba, giardia, pinworms and tapeworms. It takes about 6 weeks to remove parasites **and their eggs** from the body. Many people see complete eradication of chronic disease symptoms just from this type of cleanse.

Your healing outcome is very much dependent on you. If you give it 100% you will be giving the best possible support to your body's innate healing efforts. A one month commitment is nothing compared to years of continuous illness and far less arduous, or dangerous, than a stay in hospital, no matter how quick or convenient, it appears. The most difficult step to take, in any change, is the FIRST. What are you waiting for?

Fasting or Starving?

Confusion exists, mostly among those who have never tried it, that fasting is the same as starving. Not so. Fasting is defined as follows:

'The voluntary denial of food to a system which is diseased, and which, because of disease, does not require nourishment until rested, cleansed, and the digestive 'fire' restored. Then, and not till then, is food supplied. Then, and not till then, does starvation begin.'

Putting it simply. Fast when sick. Once cured, eat again.

What is 'digestive fire'? In Ayurveda, the concept of 'fire' (Agni) and digestion are extremely important. Without the ability to properly break down your food, nutrients cannot be assimilated. A 'fire' can burn strongly or weakly. Levels of hydrochloric acid (HCL) in the stomach can be weak or strong. Try an experiment. Wait until hungry, then consume an ice-cream or chilled drink. Your hunger will go. Why? Because you have extinguished your digestive 'fire'. If you then eat, food becomes hard to break down because the digestive fire is out.

Frozen products and iced drinks are unnatural. They cause fats to solidify, digestion to take longer, with more energy consumed. If your appetite is weak, you need to stoke the 'fire' with warming herbs and spices, not extinguish it. Supplementing with HCL supplements can make a big difference in breaking down food. As can digestive enzymes. One way to increase HCL production is to take 1tsp Apple Cider Vinegar before each meal.

When we are unwell, our bodies tell us to stop eating. We lose our appetite. However, due to addiction, habit and ignorance, we do not listen and continue to eat. We even force sick children to eat, even when they do not wish to, telling them it is to "keep your strength up".

When you eat without hunger, food becomes toxic to the body, fermenting and putrefying in the intestinal tract, producing toxins which are then taken up by the blood and deposited in other areas, such as the joints. Stress is placed upon organs, which not only have to cope with sickness but this additional burden.

When you drink freshly squeezed, organic fruit or vegetable juices, during a fast, you are not starving. You are delivering concentrated doses of nutrients to your cells. Juicing simply removes the fibre. To reduce weight loss, juice combinations can be higher in calories. The classic 'Master Cleanse' includes organic maple syrup, which provides around 400 calories per day. Increasing or decreasing the maple syrup, adjust calories. I do not recommend commercial maple syrup since it is difficult to find truly organic versions. Instead use freshly squeezed sugar-cane juice, or raw cane sugar, if it is available. In some fasts I do not use sugars at all, such as an anti-candida fast.

What caused us to be sick in the first place? A major cause of disease is impure blood. Impure blood is caused by impaired digestion from (a) Poor eating habits; (b) Incorrect food choices; (c) eating more than is needed for repair and growth of tissue cells. The resolution is to stop eating, clean up the system, reset digestion and correct eating habits. Historically, this has been done by fasting, sometimes assisted by additional treatments, such as bodywork and steam baths. The ancient Roman Baths are famous. Baden Baden, in Germany, also has wonderful mineral baths.

How Long to Fast?

Jesus fasted for 40 days and nights. Pythagoras fasted his students for 21 days, to make their minds sharper. Some fast until the tongue is clean. Others until their disease is resolved. Some take a break then repeat the fast, later.

15 years ago, the recommendation was to fast at regular intervals, such as the changing of the seasons. I recommended this myself. However, since we are taking in so many toxins, on a daily basis, that advice is somewhat inadequate. Make elimination of toxins part of your daily routine.

What Juices?

Over the years, practitioners have learned which fruit and vegetable combinations are best suited to which disorders. If you watch TV or follow celebrity juicing experts, you will be dazzled by their creativity. They do a great job but, like circus acts, tend to over-egg the pudding. They need to stay relevant, make a name for themselves and keep people interested. Some ingredients, like dairy or muesli, I would not consider suitable for healing.

Our retreats include fruit and vegetable shakes, using a wonderful array of organic fruits and vegetables, grown locally and picked fresh. For chronic disease you are better off consuming mono-juices, using nature's hard-core 'cleansers' and 'scrubbers', like black grapes and citrus. It is not easy to find uncontaminated grapes but lemons work well on a variety of conditions. Fall back on vegetable juices, or water-only fasts, if sensitive to fruit juices.

Many and varied are the possibilities. Have Candida? Try a Colloidal Silver, Apple cider vinegar or young coconut water fast. There are juices for arthritis, heart disease and cancer. Select fresh, ripe, seasonal produce. We do provide solid food in the form of fruit shakes or salads. However, liquids are preferable to solids as so many of us have compromised digestions. The ancients made it clear. In order to recover one's health, you must stop eating. Enjoy shakes AFTER you have healed.

It is important, with any fast, to start and finish gently. 24 hours prior to the fast, eat soft fruits and steamed vegetables. This reduces the burden of digestion and prepares the body for the start of the fast. Avoid dense foods. Break the fast, correctly. Eat only soft fruits, then steamed vegetables, like pumpkin, for two days after. Some believe staying completely raw is best. After not eating for 7 days or more your food will taste divine!

What is Ketosis?

Ketogenic diets are increasingly fashionable. This is not quite fasting. You basically strip carbohydrates out of the diet and burn fat. Very much like the Atkins Diet. Ketosis occurs when the body does not have enough glucose for energy. Instead stored fats are converted to glucose. Toxins and waste, released from fat stores, are then excreted. If you cannot go raw vegan, Ketogenic diets are recommended. For diabetics, in particular.

Watching the Scales

Female guests are often obsessed by the scales, worrying they are not shedding the weight they are so desperate to lose. Understand, at the start of any fast, while you may not see fat loss externally, accumulated fat **internally** (e.g. fatty liver) is being broken down and consumed. The scales may not be moving fast but you are becoming firmer and healthier. Due to retained water, body weight can fluctuate, by the hour. One snapshot isn't telling you much and may only make you anxious. We prefer you to forget the scales and concentrate on improved health.

"80% of my patients were well just after doing my thorough bowel cleansing program"
*- **Richard Schulze***

Water Cures

In his bestselling book **Your Body's Many Cries for Water,** Dr. F. Batmanghelidj (a respected, conventional medical Doctor) explains that the cause of many of today's disorders, including pain and Cancer, is chronic dehydration. In his books he provides scholarly examples of conditions cured by increasing fluid intake. One health writer had this to say about Dr. Batmanghelidj's follow-up book, **'Water Cures. Drugs Kill'**

"...after a wake-up call to America and Britain, Dr. B outlines several disease states (warning symptoms) which progress to actual damage. He elaborates multiple and varied case histories which confirm dehydration as the cause of symptoms. His examples are so varied that almost anyone could find, within the pages of his books, information directly relevant to his/her personal situation."

The message we receive from Dr. Batmanghelidj is you are not only what you eat (I might add 'what your cells assimilate') but also what you drink. Since water is assimilated easily and rapidly, and costs only pennies, it is the perfect treatment.

Do you drink water? You will be surprised at the number who don't. When asked why, the answer most give is, they do not like the taste. I sympathize. Municipal and bottled waters do not taste clean because they aren't. There are no glaciers in my area. Nor running, dancing, gurgling mineral springs. If there were, a drinks giant has already stuck a bottling plant on it.

It seems like we have little choice but to pay outrageous prices, for that which nature provides us, free. Little realizing the higher price we pay in diminished health. Think about mineral or spring water. What kind of minerals do they contain? Not what you might think. They are the magnesium and calcium and iron found in dissolved rocks. If I could absorb iron from sucking a rusty nail, I would do so. But that's not how nature works. **Inorganic** minerals cannot be absorbed or utilized by our cells. Only **organic** minerals, which nature provides us, already filtered by plants, can be assimilated. The consequence of drinking crushed or dissolved rocks, is the gradual accumulation of pounds of inorganic matter in our filters... kidneys, liver, joints and tissues... contributing to, or directly causing, disease. This is why water cures are a great place to start and why clearing the kidneys and achieving proper kidney filtration is the goal of many holistic practitioners. Water is the best solvent there is but it needs to be the **right** water. Distilled water, having no dissolved solids, picks up and either dissolves, or excretes, accumulated matter. The junk we can't currently flush away because we aren't hydrated enough. Many of us are dehydrated, do not know it, nor realize how many disorders are caused by a lack of sufficient water. Our bodies are made up of water:

Muscles 75%.
Blood 82%.
Lungs 90%.
Brain 76%.
Bones 25%.

Detox programs resolve many disorders because water and juices hydrate the tissues. Remember the sponge analogy? Place a dirty sponge in a bucket of water overnight and in the morning the sponge is clean with the dirt lying on the bottom. What would happen if there were insufficient water in the bucket? The sponge would stay dirty. Likewise, our bodies. Not drinking sufficient water restricts the lymphatic system's ability to mobilize waste, and transport it to the organs of elimination.

Protocol 1

Drink 1½ litres of distilled water, on an empty stomach, first thing in the morning. Do not eat or drink for the following hour. Do this 3x daily, for 1 week, for arthritis and rheumatism, then 2x daily until you are healed. For all other disorders, 2x daily is recommended.

Protocol 2

Dr Batmanghelidj's Method is to drink 8 glasses of water per day, with ½ teaspoon of sea salt. 1/8th teaspoon of sea salt to each 8oz glass. (Use uniodized sea salt or Celtic sea salt.)

If too little water makes me sick, won't too much? Yes. Water fast until the body is clean and/or your disease condition resolved. If you have difficulty increasing fluid intake, build up slowly or drink water throughout the day.

Frank Tippett

Frank Tippett was diagnosed with Multiple Sclerosis (MS) in April 2000. MRIs showed the myelin sheath missing and plaque on the brain. Frank suffered numbness, tingling, pain, slurred speech, a loss of control of his right arm, walking and balance problems, his bodily functions slowed down and he was constantly tired.

The doctor put Frank on Avonex, which helped for three days out of the week. This became more as soon as Frank commenced his Water Cure. He also took cold-pressed flax seed oil, B Complex, lecithin, a one-a-day vitamin, and potassium. Two and a half months later Frank's numbness and tingling were gone. In the following months his walking and balance improved and bodily functions returned to normal.

In December 2001 Frank came off the Avonex. All the tests for MS showed he was in excellent health. As an added bonus, Frank had an enlarged prostate for seven years. His family doctor checked it during his last visit. It was normal.

Frank feels to deal with the effects of MS you need a positive attitude, open mind and a willingness to try other treatments.

"I haven't felt this good in twenty years", says Frank. "Thanks to Dr. Batmanghelidj".

A Most Unexpected Cure

I must have a mischievous streak. With all the possibilities to choose from, I pick the sensational.

'Urine therapy' is an ancient healing practice that has fallen out of favour in the last 150 years. Well, almost. You may be surprised to learn urine is still used, medicinally, today. Urine is an ingredient in a number of products, such as face cream. Its origin disguised using innocent-sounding labels. In Ayurveda they call urine, 'Shivambu Shastra' which means "Water of Shiva", a very auspicious name. There is even an annual **World Conference on Urine Therapy**, attended by scholars.

Have you ever tasted or drank your own urine? "Yuck!" I hear you say. Why would anyone drink their own urine? It is a waste product, surely? Dirty, smelly and dangerous.

Why would I even consider drinking my own urine? Well, desperation, mostly, and curiosity. Frustrated with failure to recover from my illness, I came across a book with a remarkable story to tell. **'Your Own Perfect Medicine'** by Martha Christy.

The following is from Biomedx:

'Ms. Christy was sick. Very sick. For a very long time. Pelvic inflammatory disease, ulcerative colitis, Chron's disease, chronic fatigue syndrome, Hashimoto's disease, mononucleosis. She had severe kidney infections, two miscarriages, chronic cystitis, severe candida, endometriosis, adrenal insufficiency, serious chronic ear and sinus infections, food and chemical allergies. And that wasn't the half of it. She had every conceivable medical test, her share of surgery, and drugs – plenty of them. Then she tried all forms of alternative therapy. Homeopathy, herbs, mega-vitamins and liv-cell treatments in Mexico. After traditional medicine failed to work, she and her husband spent over $100,000 trying to get her well with alternative approaches. Nothing worked.

And then one day, her husband brought home a little book that told of how individuals had been cured of even the worst diseases with a seemingly strange and little-known natural therapy. Soon afterwards, she began the therapy herself. From the first day she began, she received almost instantaneous relief from her incurable constipation and fluid retention. Within a week, her severe abdominal and pelvic pain was gone.

The chronic cystitis and yeast infections (internal and external) soon disappeared and her food allergies, exhaustion, and digestive problems all began to heal.

After a few more months, her colds, flu, sore throats and on again, off again viral symptoms disappeared. Her hair which had fallen out by the handfuls after her fifth surgery became thick and lustrous. Her weight normalized, and her energy and strength came back. After nearly 30 years of non-stop illness, Martha Christy was whole again.'

The incredible 'Miracle Cure' Martha Christy discovered?

Her urine.

Let's get the main objection out of the way. The smell. If your diet is healthy, your output won't smell like a public toilet in an Irish bar. It will have virtually no scent, taste, and runs almost clear. *"A hint of summer meadows"* I used to joke with friends.

Urine is not what we think it is. In her book, Martha explains:

"Urine is not, as many believe, the excess water from food and liquids that goes through the intestines and is ejected from the body as "waste". It is much different and much more. When you eat, the food you ingest is eventually broken down in the stomach and intestines into extremely small molecules. These molecules are absorbed into tiny tubules in the intestinal wall and then pass through these tubes into the blood stream.

The blood circulates throughout your body carrying these food molecules and other nutrients, along with critical immune defense and regulating elements such as red and white blood cells, antibodies, plasma, microscopic proteins, hormones, enzymes, etc., which are all manufactured at different locations in the body.

As the blood circulates, it passes through the liver where toxins are removed and later excreted from the body in the form of solid waste. Eventually, this now purified "cleaned" blood makes its way to the kidneys. When blood enters the kidneys it is filtered through an immensely complex and intricate system of minute tubules called nephron through which the blood is literally "squeezed" at high pressure. This filtering process removes excess amounts of water, salts and other elements in the blood that your body does not need at the time.

These excess elements are collected within the kidney in the form of a purified, sterile, watery solution called urine. Many of the constituents of this filtered watery solution, or urine, are then reabsorbed by the nephron and delivered back into the bloodstream. The remainder of the urine passes out of the kidneys into the bladder and is then excreted from the body.

The function of the kidneys is to keep the various elements in your blood balanced. When your body doesn't need something at a particular time, it is excreted – not because it is toxic or poisonous or bad for the body, but simply because the body does not need that particular element at the time.

Medical researchers have discovered that many of the elements of the blood that are found in urine have enormous medicinal value, and when reintroduced to the body, they boost the body's immune defences and stimulate healing in a way that nothing else does".

Having read her story, what struck me most about Martha's experience was the terrible ordeal she went through. Both modern and alternative medicine failed to help her. Thanks to this ancient healing knowledge, Martha's 30-year struggle finally ended.

Martha doesn't just present one anecdote about her own experience. She hired a research firm to search the scientific and medical literature. Her book is filled with references and research findings.

In 1954, Greek physician, **Dr. Evangelos Danopoulos**, reported urine had anticancer properties. As did German Doctor **Hans Nieper**, who reportedly cured Ronald Reagan of colon cancer and used urea in one of his formulas.

I hope you are motivated to investigate this totally misunderstood, natural healing substance for yourself. If on a budget, isn't it worth a try? It is FREE. If you have tried everything else and nothing has worked, what have you got to lose? Cleaning up your diet will remove any unpleasant taste and smell. If it doesn't, then mix with fruit juice, or take as a homeopathic preparation, where there is no smell or taste at all.

You may not realize it but you may already be absorbing someone else's urine into your cells. **Pergonal** is a fertility drug made from human urine. **Urokinase**, a urine ingredient, is sold as a blood clot dissolver for unblocking coronary arteries. Urea, medically proven to be one of the best moisturizers in the world, is packaged in expensive creams and lotions. Take the M out of **Murine** eye drops and what do you have?

Some cannot do it no matter how dire their situation. Some victims, trapped in building collapses, or lost at sea, survived by drinking their own urine. The ones who did not, died. The movie '127 hours' is the incredible, true story of **Aron Ralston**, who cut off his arm and drank his own urine to survive after being trapped 20 miles from civilization. Aron said drinking his own urine had been harder, psychologically, than cutting off his arm. Psychological squeamishness is not confined to urine. I am squeamish myself when I see northern village Thais tucking into roasted bugs and beetles. Could I eat them if my life depended on it? I hope I am never put to the test!

Beginning to understand urine is not harmful, is a potential 'cure-all' and might be a life-saver? Claims urine can cure over 175 different diseases come from personal testimonies.

The following is a suggested routine.

Day 1. 1-5 drops (of morning, mid-stream urine)

Day 2. 5-10 drops in the morning.

Day 3. 5-10 drops in the morning and evening.

Gradually increase the amount as needed, to obtain results for your condition. Work up to drinking an ounce or two at a time. Oh yes. Expect to get ribbed by others. Treat it with a little humour. We are far too serious. And let me know how the 'amber nectar' works for you.

"Bottoms up!"

Reversing Diabetes

Dr Gabriel Cousens, at the Tree of Life Center, Arizona, has shown, for over 30 years, Type 2 Diabetes can be reversed. Dr Cousens tells us Type 2 Diabetes is one of the easiest disorders to resolve because Type 2 Diabetes is a LIFESTYLE disease. Caused by what we are putting in our mouths. His nutritional approach has mainstream support, following the 2011 UK **Newcastle Study** ([15](#))

On the Newcastle Study diet, it took 8 weeks to restore health. The program involved adopting a strict 600-calorie per day intake. Study participants were Type IIs who had diabetes for at least 4 years. The basic idea was to try and mimic the results of gastric bypass surgery.

There is nothing particularly complicated or unique about the Newcastle Study. It is simply a reduced-calorie diet that attempts to switch you over from carb-burning to fat-burning. When you switch to fat-burning the body will use the fat around your organs FIRST. This is what the Ketogenic Diet does. Those who stuck to the diet successfully restored pancreatic function, after losing a lot of weight.

Keep in mind, for all disorders, including diabetes, we apply the **First and Second Laws of Health**.

1. STOP doing whatever is making you sick.

2. Do the opposite. Instead of eating insulin-producing foods, eat insulin-reducing foods/foods that do not trigger an insulin response.

As you are probably tired of hearing, making lifestyle changes is almost impossible without support. 8 weeks is tough, which is why I created our **Reverse Diabetes** retreat and **Reverse Diabetes at Home** health coaching programs. Results are rapid. Blood sugar normalizes within 4 days and complete reversal is achieved within 21 days for approximately 88% of retreat guests. With a little more time the other 12% will get there too. The retreat works quickly because the program is focussed. You can't tip-toe downstairs to raid the fridge for that week-old, stale donut you can't bear to toss in the bin.

Dr Cousens recently incorporated juice-fasting into his protocol. Previously it was raw food. I have always preferred juicing, to eating, as it works faster and is easier to stick to. This appears to defy logic but think about it. When eating salads I find people are left un-satiated and are constantly hungry. On juices, after 36-48 hours, your body switches over to fasting mode. Your digestion 'switches off'. No hunger. You can go without food for 10, 20, 30 days, with ease.

Using cleansing, bodywork, herbs, hydrotherapy, and Ayurvedic methods, fasting blood sugar normalizes within 1-4 days, excess fat is cleared from the liver and pancreatic function restored. Dr Cousens has done a great service to the world by showing us the way. His methods are classical natural healing.

What about pre-diabetes?

Hypoglycaemia, Hyperglycaemia and Metabolic Disorder (Syndrome X) fall into a category called 'prediabetes'.

Hypoglycaemia is a condition that results from low blood sugar. Symptoms of hypoglycaemia can include food cravings, weakness, depression, insomnia and more. Many people treat hypoglycemia with sweets, biscuits, potato chips, chocolate, etc… to raise their sugar level quickly. This works – but only for a short period. When you take in food, high in carbohydrates, or sugar, your body will sense a sharp increase in your blood sugar level. As a result, the pancreas produces high amounts of insulin and your sugar level plummets. The drop triggers sugar cravings and you repeat the experience. Again and again and again. Until your pancreas is worn-out and you become insulin-dependent.

'Yo-yoing' like this, is harmful and unnecessary.

Cure rate for prediabetes?

100% within 14 days.

Carlos Cervantes

In July 2008 Carlos Cervantes was diagnosed with Type II Diabetes. His fasting blood sugar was over 500 (28 mmol/l) and he was experiencing thirst, constant tiredness and was semi-comatose. Metformin caused him to gain 30lbs, so he switched to Glipizide, where he gained another 5lbs.

In 2010, after 6 months of a diabetic-driven ear infection, Carlos was put on insulin. In December he developed his first diabetic foot ulcer, then a second, in June 2011, so serious he faced amputation. There were problems with his kidneys, liver and eyesight, and painful neuropathy in his feet. In Feb 2011 Carlos had a heart attack. 3 months later his insulin was increased by his Doctor. By this point, Carlos accepted he was going to die.

A higher power had other ideas and 3 hours later, Carlos was drawn to a 2-minute news item that completely turned him around. It was about the Newcastle University Study. During the study, a group of Type 2 diabetics, led by Professor Roy Taylor, completely reversed their diabetes within 8 weeks, on a reduced-calorie diet and exercise.

Carlos decided to try the diet but instead of 800 calories per day, he opted for 600, for 64 days. Carlos found it tough. But, to his credit, was very determined, consuming soups, salads, lots of water and a little gentle walking.

On the 18th of July 2011, the day after starting the program, Carlos stopped his insulin completely. Within 11 days his blood sugar readings were normal.

Today, Carlos is healthy. His blood sugar levels range from 67-73 (approx. 3.7 mmol/l) and all his diabetic symptoms have gone. He weighs 174 lbs, dramatically down from a high of 305 lbs.

30 Days to Health

The **30 Days to Health** program has been used to save the lives of thousands of extremely sick people. It incorporates classical naturopathic steps. You may not need all 30 days, or you may need more. We don't all respond in the same way. Success depends on how well you apply yourself and the nature of your disorder.

The program attacks the disease process in a sustained way and keeps attacking it, until resolved. It is designed to achieve quick results. You can progress more slowly, with a raw vegan or vegetarian diet. These work too. However, the longer the timescale, the greater chance of self-sabotage. As 84-year old Dan said:

"There are quick, medium and slow ways to restore health. All have their advantages and disadvantages. It seemed preferable, at least to me, that if I am going to forego all my treats in order to restore my health, I would rather get it over and done with quickly."

On the program you are going to:

1. Commit 100% to the program

2. Stop whatever you are doing that is making you sick, and reverse it (Laws of Similars & Opposites)

3. Ensure your channels of elimination are open

4. Clear physical, emotional, psychological, energetic and spiritual blockages – **The 5 Layers of Healing**.

5. Move your blood and lymph

6. Balance your PH

7. Improve cellular respiration (ensure oxygen is getting to your cells)

8. Flood your body with nutrients

Do the program alone or seek a professional to support you. Bear in mind this is the full program, based on not knowing the cause of your disorder(s). If you know the cause, you may require just a thorough bowel cleanse. Stick with it because by the time you are finished, you are going to feel transformed.

Assuming steps 1&2 are actioned:

Step 3. Ensure the channels of elimination (bowels, lungs, liver, kidneys and skin) are open.

The bowels need to be moving and emptied. This can be done with laxative teas like Senna; Castor Oil, Triphala (an herb), salt water flushes (using uniodized sea salt), or enemas. Enema kits can be bought in most pharmacies or health stores. Dr Richard Schulze' online herbal store sells two intestinal formulas. The first is to get the bowels moving. If your bowels are moving okay (many people are constipated) you do not need it. The second assists in cleansing and restoring the colon.

Breathing exercises strengthen and expand the lungs, get you breathing properly and bring in more oxygen, while expelling carbonic acid and other harmful wastes, stagnating at the bottom of your lungs. Flushes will eliminate toxins from liver, gall bladder and kidneys. Dry and wet skin-brushing clears blocked pores and gets your circulation and lymph moving.

Step 4. Clear physical, emotional, psychological, energetic and spiritual blockages. Cleanse with juices and address the 5 Layers. Review the chapters on **EFT+NLP** and **Breaking The Chains**. These techniques are easy to learn and apply, yourself, at home.

Step 5. Move blood and lymph with massage, contrast bathing and exercise.

Step 6. Balance your PH. Use fruit and vegetable juices to alkalize tissues and flush acid wastes.

Step 7. Provide proper cellular respiration with chlorophyll, exercise, breathing exercises. 3% Hydrogen Peroxide drops not only oxidize pathogens (our body produces hydrogen peroxide to kill rogue cells) but bring more oxygen to cells. Ed McCabe's book **Flood Your Body with Oxygen** is a good resource.

Step 8. It is hard to consume sufficient vegetable matter, in its raw state, to obtain all the nutrients. You may not have enough digestive 'fire' to break down vegetable fibres. Juicing allows nutrients to be absorbed rapidly. Moringa is a complete source of vitamins, minerals and amino acids.

The following is an example **Daily Schedule** I use during retreats. Juices and herbs can be selected to address specific conditions. Explanations for each task are provided.

TIME	DAILY SCHEDULE
0600	On rising, greet the day positively. Open arms wide and say "I FEEEEEEEL GREEEAAATTTT!!!"
0605	Dry Skin Brushing + beat yourself up! + Hot & Cold Shower (1 min Hot, 1 min Cold. 7x)
0630	Lemon, Chili, Sugar Cane Juice + Tincture
0700	Morning walk + deep breathing. Or swim + Pranayama in fresh morning air + stretching/Yoga
0800	Salt Water flush or 'Mae West' retention enema
0900	Lemon, Chili, Sugar Cane Juice + Tincture + Bentonite Shake
0905	Sun and wind-bathing with Coconut/Sesame Oil
1000	Herbal Steam Sauna (20-30mins) followed by Ice water dip or shower. Skin brush + vigorous rub with towel. Potassium Broth
1030	Sesame Oil Massage + Deep Reflexology + Hot Herbal Bolus
1100	Lemon, Chili, Sugar Cane Juice + Tincture + Bentonite Shake
1500	Lemon, Chili, Sugar Cane Juice + Tincture + Bentonite Shake
1600	Sun + wind-bathing with Coconut/Sesame Oil + drink water
1700	Potassium Broth + 30 minute walk, swim or Yoga. Breathe hard and encourage sweating.
1930	Lemon, Chili, Sugar Cane Juice + Tincture + Bentonite Shake
2000	Relax

Start the Day in the Right Way

Waking up grumpy? Go to your bedroom window, throw open the curtains and shout out loudly,

"I FEEEEEEEL GREEEAAATTTT!!!"

Fake it until you make it. Do this every morning. Some days you can't do it. Never mind. Switch off, shut down, do nothing and tell yourself,

"It's only a passing cloud".

Juicing

The simplest and most famous juice for detoxing comes from 'The Master Cleanse'. Drink 8oz every hour or 16oz, every 2 hours. Make up drinks, to go, if you are out for any length of time.

- Juice of one lemon,
- Pinch of chilli powder
- Organic maple syrup or fresh sugar cane juice (to taste).

Lemon Soda - a great way to start the day
- Juice of 1 lemon
- ¼ tsp of baking soda

Combine in 8oz of water and drink. A pinch of chilli powder will dilate blood vessels and assist in delivering cleansing and healing factors around your body. Drinking it hot is also beneficial. Cold or ice drinks shock the digestive system, put out the digestive fire and solidify fats... the opposite of what you are aiming for. We need fats and fluids to flow smoothly, in the same way warm oil does in a car.

Drink water in between juices. Keep those cells hydrated.

Dry Skin Brushing

Brush your skin before you bath or shower. This stimulates the neuro-muscular system (invigorates you), improves blood circulation and stagnation in the lymphatic system and sloughs off dead skin. Use a loofah or firm (not too stiff) brush. Brush toward the heart.

Beat Yourself Up!

Using the knuckles of your clenched fist, 'tap-tap-tap' all over your body. The idea is to break up and dislodge 'dirt' and blockages, as well as stimulate circulation. Ask your partner to 'beat you up', or do the program together and beat each other up! It is a great way to bond. No bruising, please!

Herbal Steam Sauna

Herbal steam saunas enhance detoxification. At Antarana, we include 10 different herbs and sometimes ozone. Neither are strictly necessary, just as long as you are sweating. Different Constitutional Types need different lengths of time in the sauna. Slim 'Air' types stay a maximum of 15 minutes. Medium-build, 'Fire' types, also 15 minutes (they get too heated). Heavy 'Earth' and 'Water' types up to 30 minutes. When you exit, douse yourself, or have a dip in cold water, to close the pores. Scandinavians have used saunas for detoxification for centuries.

Note: We do not recommend FAR Infra-Red Saunas. Almost all models have been found to emit unacceptable levels of radiation.

Breathing (Pranayama)

In Yoga, many different breathing exercises exist. I am a huge fan of Bhastrika (The Bellows Breath) and Kapalbhati (Skull Polishing Breath). Aniloma Viloma (Alternate Nostril Breathing) balances the sympathetic and parasympathetic nervous system, as well as improves relaxation and oxygenation. Deep breath any time you are outside. Fresh air will help you heal faster.

*Search for these names and instructional videos on YouTube.

Sunbathing (Heliotherapy)

Every day (privacy permitting) strip naked and take a sun and air bath for a maximum of one hour, when the sun is weak. In 'Nature Cure' centres, they apply organic, extra virgin coconut oil to leg ulcers, varicose veins and skin conditions like eczema and psoriasis, with excellent results. You can also use organic Sesame oil (from black seeds). If you cannot remove your clothes, apply oil to bare legs. Do not use sun creams, they are toxic. DO NOT BURN.

Sesame Oil

Sesame oil is immensely popular in India. It is a favourite oil for massage, as it penetrates the skin easily, nourishing and detoxifying even the deepest tissue layers. Used regularly, sesame oil is wonderful for reducing stress and tension, nourishing the nervous system and preventing nervous disorders, relieving fatigue and insomnia, while promoting strength and vitality.

Regular oiling restores moisture to the skin, keeping it soft, flexible and young looking. It lubricates the body internally, particularly joints and bowels, and eases symptoms of dryness such as irritating coughs, cracking joints and hard stools. Sesame oil massage helps calm babies, lulls them to sleep and improves growth of the brain and the nervous system. Its antioxidants slow the aging process and promote longevity.

Massage and Oil

Massage oils and wet heat help loosen and liquefy toxins and humors in the skin and blood (called the outer disease pathway), dislodging and removing the heavy, sticky toxins from the smallest channels. Thus, toxins can begin to drain from the central disease pathway (deeper tissues) and flow into the GI tract. Secretions are also activated, enabling easier transport of toxins and wastes as they return to the GI tract for elimination. Oil lubricates and protects tissues from damage, as toxins return.

Finally, since Vata (air) is responsible for movement, oil lubrication restores proper Vata functioning, allowing for proper flowing of wastes and toxins to removal sites. Classical oils to use are Sesame and Castor Oil. Oils can be infused with herbs but this is not required for your DIY program.

Reflexology

Having an expert massage your lower legs and feet is a treat. An authentic Reflexology session can help identify problems in the body and is very relaxing. Some practitioners use strong pressure to break up crystalline formations. This can be painful. The less painful way is to dissolve crystal formation by alkalyzing the tissues or applying the Borax protocol.

Bowel Cleansing

Flush the bowels at the start of, and during a cleanse. Flush the entire gastro-intestinal tract by drinking 1.5-2lts of salt water, commencing after 7am. Consume within 40 minutes.

Most people manage a salt water flush without difficulty. However, if you are particularly toxic, you can feel a little nauseous and may vomit. If so, good! It cleanses the stomach. Any nausea clears quickly.

Ensure you put in sufficient salt. Salt alters the specific gravity of water, making the body think it is food (not liquid) and, thus, directs salt water into the bowel, instead of kidneys. Use 1 level tablespoon of sea salt in 2lt clean water. If this does not work, increase the amount of salt. It will do no harm. If for some reason salt water cannot be taken, drink a laxative tea, morning and evening, until bowels are clear.

'Mae West' Retention Enema

The Master Cleanse recommends salt water flushes (SWF) each morning. However, some find drinking salt water too difficult. If this is you, try one SWF on the first morning then switch to a daily 'Mae West' enema. This has three ingredients. Organic coffee, sea salt and baking soda, in 2lt of clean water. Organic coffee stimulates the liver. Sea Salt is cleansing and mineral-rich. Baking soda softens and alkalizes the water. Some people use Colema boards or special colon-cleansing machines but an enema kit, with a 2-litre bag, is inexpensive and works fine.

1. Put 2 tablespoons of organic coffee in a percolator or boil in a stainless steel pan, in 8-16oz of water.

2. Once boiled, allow to cool a little, add 1 tablespoon each of sea salt and baking soda (aluminium-free).

3. Top up to 2 lts with water. Pour into your enema bag.

4. Empty half the contents of the enema bag into your colon (instructions come with the kit). You will feel the need to evacuate. Go ahead and do so, then empty the rest of the liquid, in the enema bag, into your colon. Try to retain for 15 minutes. If you feel cramping, take deep breaths, until the cramps ease.

Note: Salt water will flush the whole GI tract, while an enema only flushes the lower part of the colon.

Bentonite Shake

Bentonite & Psyllium mixtures are like taking a broom to intestinal walls. They attract and soak up released toxins as well as pull fecal matter off colon walls. Taking this is important during the initial few days, when levels of circulating toxins are high. I make my own but you can buy Dr Schulze Intestinal Formula #2 (16)

(I have no affiliation with providers). Here is what the supplier site says:

'Intestinal Formula #2 contains the three most powerful and effective absorbers and neutralizers known: clay, charcoal and pectin.

Our Bentonite Clay will actually absorb up to 40 times its weight in intestinal faecal matter and waste. It also smothers and draws out all types of intestinal parasites. Activated Willow Charcoal is the greatest absorbing agent for every toxin and poison known. It will absorb and render harmless over 3,000 known drug residues, pesticides, insecticides and just about every harmful chemical. This is why it is the active ingredient in nearly every water filter made today. Apple Pectin draws numerous harmful substances out of your intestines, especially heavy metals like mercury and lead and carcinogenic radioactive materials.

The addition of Marshmallow Root, along with Psyllium Seed and Flax Seed, makes the formula mucilaginous. Mucilaginous means all the water and herbs can sit in your bowel, soaking against the internal wall of your colon, softening and breaking up old, dried and hardened fecal waste that may have been in you for years.'

It is called a shake because you mix the powder with water (or fruit juice), shake it vigorously, then drink. Wash it down with clean, fresh water.

Potassium Broth

Potassium broth will flush your system of unwanted salts and acids while providing a concentrated amount of vitamins and minerals. It is a great immune booster.

Ingredients
4 bulbs garlic
2 large onions – peeled
1 bunch chopped kale
1 stick chopped celery
5 pounds chopped carrots
5 pounds potatoes (peels only)
3 beets with greens (peels only)
4 chopped jalapeños
1 bunch organic parsley
4 quarts distilled water

Fill your pot with the chopped vegetables. Cover with distilled or reverse osmosis water and simmer for 1 hour. Add water as needed to keep vegetables covered. Strain, then refrigerate what is not immediately needed. Spread over 2-3 days.

Additional Routines

Every day take a walk outside in your bare feet and shuffle them in the grass, or dirt, even lie down on the earth. Use only natural soaps, shampoos and toothpastes. Never use any deodorants, perfumes, colognes, etc. You may use pure herbal essential oils, if you smell. Wear only natural fibre clothing, cotton, wool and silk. No polyester, nylon or even blends.

Liver & Gallbladder Cleanse

The health of the liver is crucial to long-term health. A congested liver is the reason behind many modern diseases such as acne, yeast infection, leaky gut, etc. Doctors have found, in almost all cancer patients, the condition of the liver was extremely poor.

An overload of toxins causes a congested liver. Toxins eventually circulate back into your bloodstream, where they can end up anywhere – joints, brain, heart or other organs. Your kidneys become burdened by the extra workload, which contributes to a vicious cycle. If your colon is clogged, as well, the liver has an even tougher time eliminating toxins. A congested liver, like a clogged colon, is caused by a poor diet of refined carbohydrates, hydrogenated fats, preservatives, foods laced with hormones, environmental pollutants, overuse of antibiotics, drugs, and stress.

You already do a gall bladder flush many times a week without realizing. Eating fat and protein triggers the gallbladder to empty after twenty minutes. The stored bile makes its trip down the common bile duct to the intestine. All we are doing is triggering the same process in an optimal way. The difference is, your bowels will be fully empty and bile ducts relaxed, due to the magnesium in the Epsom Salts, which acts as both a laxative and muscle relaxant. Oil triggers the gall bladder to empty itself of bile (and anything else in there) and lemon juice helps move the oil along.

Cholesterol & Bile

We do not need cholesterol from our diet. The liver produces all the cholesterol we need. The liver also produces bile, a greenish-brown fluid, charged with the significant responsibility of digesting fats. Bile is sent to the gallbladder, where it is concentrated and stored. When you eat, the gallbladder contracts and releases stored bile, where it helps break down any fat in your food. If the bile within your gallbladder becomes chemically unbalanced, it can form into hardened particles that eventually form stones.

Gallstones

Many statements are made by alternative practitioners to the effect that a liver and gall bladder flush removes gallstones. Our research shows this is true only for some people, with smaller stones and 'chaff' being ejected. Images of thousands of small green 'stones' one sees, online, are formed by the olive oil/lemon juice mixture.

'About 1 in 12 people have gallstones and may be unaware of it. As the stones grow and become more numerous the back pressure on the liver causes it to make less bile. It is also thought to slow the flow of lymphatic fluid. Imagine the situation if your garden hose had marbles in it. Much less water would flow, which in turn would decrease the ability of the hose to squirt out the marbles. With gallstones, much less cholesterol leaves the body, and cholesterol levels may rise. Gallstones, being porous, can pick up all the bacteria, cysts, viruses and parasites that are passing through the liver. In this way "nests" of infection are formed, forever supplying the body with fresh bacteria and parasite stages. No stomach infection such as ulcers or intestinal bloating can be cured permanently without removing these gallstones from the liver.' – **Dr Hulda Clark**

Our aim is not primarily to remove gallstones (we are pleased when we don't see any) but to clear the liver and gall bladder of toxins, during and after a fast. Flushes also improve overall health. Some people have experienced relief from allergies, bursitis, back pain and other conditions after a liver flush. More so with repeated flushes. If you don't see any stones, be happy. If you ever get a larger stone, you will know about it.

Toxins & Parasites

Anyone conducting a lengthy fast will have parasites dying off from around day 7. Toxins, from the detox, are also being eliminated. The liver, being the most important organ of elimination, has to work hard to remove this waste from the body. A liver flush opens up the liver and gall bladder ducts, allowing parasites and fungi to be eliminated more easily. The free flow of bile from the liver/gall bladder will also prevent new parasite infection.

Questions of Safety

Research and feedback, after millions of flushes, shows this process to be very safe, with only 1 negative incident in 800 reported. The recipe for the flush is hundreds of years old. It involves drinking Epsom salts, followed by an olive oil and lemon juice mix, before retiring. Some have found drinking this difficult, particularly the Epsom Salts. It is easier, mixed with apple or grapefruit juice.

Epsom Salts can trigger diarrhoea but not for everyone, since the bowels are already empty after a week or more of fasting. You want the bowel empty for the flush anyway. Expect diarrhoea, a restless night and a little nausea but this quickly wears off.

'Cold Sheet' Treatment

The Cold Sheet treatment requires two people and is not for the faint-hearted. How does it work? Thanks go to my Naturopath friend, Paul Blake, for this explanation:

'In ancient Europe in a small village during the dead of winter a fever had struck the local people and many had died. One night a man who had this fever thought he would try to make it to the local doctors for treatment. So he set out on foot through the heavy snow to the doctor's house, many miles away. Before long it started to snow then turned into a blizzard. The man, sick and cold, pushed on.

Soon, in the dark, he came to a fairly wide stream with a fallen log bridge for crossing. In trying to cross the stream the man slipped, fell into the freezing water and was drenched. As he dragged himself out of the icy water he realized he was going to die before he could make it to the doctor. So he turned around hoping to make it back home to his family and at least see them one last time. He was stumbling and delirious by the time he arrived. They tucked him into bed as best they could, expecting him to die.

By the morning he had fully recovered; in fact he had not felt this good in years. Even his lumbago was gone. From then on, whenever the man was sick, he would go back to the stream and throw himself in. Well this story got out and spread across Europe and people everywhere from the common man to Kings and Queens were putting themselves through various forms of icy cold and hot treatments to cure their diseases.

From this experience, Hydrotherapy began and the Cold Sheet Treatment was born. At one time hydrotherapy was taught at all medical universities but it was sadly set aside to be replaced by drug therapy. Fortunately, for you and me, naturopathic doctors like Dr. John Ray Christopher knew better and held on to the treatment because it worked!'

Purpose

The purpose of the Cold Sheet Treatment is to artificially increase the body's temperature, thereby accelerating the body's immune response.

The important thing to remember is to keep well hydrated. A high temperature, in a well-hydrated body, is not dangerous. The temperature can rise to 103 or 104 degrees Fahrenheit. If the body is dehydrated, the body can overheat, causing seizure or damage. Drinking plenty of fluids means drinking until your stomach is full and then drinking some more. As Dr. Christopher would say, "When the tea flows out of your ears, that is enough".

Contraindications: Do not use with small children, the very elderly, heart disease or moderate-to-severe hypertensive conditions, extreme weakness and debility. This procedure is quite rigorous. If you aren't sure, do not use it.

Instructions

Begin with a cool enema of herbal tea. Red Raspberry or Catnip herbal tea is good. This is designed to cleanse and clear the bowel of loose faecal matter in preparation for step 2 the garlic injection. You may want to evacuate the bowel a couple of times. Each time hold the water in the bowel as long as you can before releasing. Be sure and lubricate the enema tip with oil.

Next use a rectal syringe from the drug store to introduce a garlic solution. In a blender mix 8-10 cloves of fresh garlic in 1 cup of water and 1 cup of apple cider vinegar. Filter out garlic pulp and save for step 4 then put the solution in the syringe. For many this is the most intense part of this procedure. It is very safe, but does burn. Squirt in as much of the solution as you can. Keep the garlic solution in as long as you can, usually about 2 minutes before expelling. Even after expelling it, you will retain enough to do you good. The burning and cramping will subside in a couple of minutes.

Make a tea bag out of a sock and add into it 1oz each of Ginger powder, Yellow Mustard powder and Cayenne Pepper powder. Fill the bath as hot as is tolerable without burning the skin and place the sock tea bag in the water. Before the patient gets in, it is important to coat the genitals with plenty of Vaseline. Put the patient in the bath and begin giving them hot/warm herbal tea to drink. Use yarrow (one of the best diaphoretics) or peppermint or ginger tea. The goal is to drink 6-8 full cups of tea. It is the helpers' job to get as much tea as possible into the patient. If the patient becomes faint or light-headed, place a cold washcloth on the forehead. Cayenne tincture in the mouth will also prevent faintness. If the muscles become rigid, or begin to spasm, use Lobelia tincture orally. Keep the patient in the tub for at least 30 minutes. Usually by 20 minutes they'll be aching to get out but keep them in as long as possible, drinking tea until, as mentioned, it is coming out their ears.

Prepare a double sized cotton sheet (it must be 100% cotton) by soaking it in a sink or tub of water and ice. Use lots of ice. Prepare the patients bed by putting a plastic sheet or lining against the mattress under the bed sheets. When the patient stands up, out of the bath, wrap the ice-cold sheet around him/her. Then escort them to bed, wrapped in the sheet. Tuck them into bed, sheet and all, then cover with natural fibre blankets. Wrap them up in a cosy cocoon with a towel around the head leaving a face opening. Dr. Christopher recommends coating the soles of the feet with a thick garlic paste, then putting socks on the feet before putting them in bed. The paste is made by mixing mashed garlic with Vaseline. You can use the garlic that you strained from step two. By lying in the sheet for several hours (preferably overnight), the body will continue to sweat out toxins. Often the sheet will be stained with these toxins. Keep the patient in bed for at least 2-3 hours, preferably all night.

Upon arising, sponge off with Apple Cider Vinegar and water (half and half) before taking a shower. This will wipe the toxins off the skin so they won't be reabsorbed during the shower.

Give the patient only fruit or vegetable juices and herbal teas, for the next 1 to 3 days, to provide a more thorough cleansing. You should continue taking immune boosting herbs and herbal formula such as Echinacea, Goldenseal, Cats Claw, Immune Boost or Anti-Plague Formula.

Modifications to the Cold Sheet Treatment

There are countless modifications to this procedure. For example with a child, you can simply put them in a warm bath, have them drink some herbal tea, give them an Immune herb, like Echinacea, then tuck them into bed. However, for the full impact and benefit, especially when it is life or death, follow the full procedure (Dr Schulze says not to weaken on the enemas or the cold sheet because it seems too radical).

When to Stop a Fast

Dr. Edward Dewey believed you should stop fasting when there is no coating on the tongue. If you check your tongue first thing in the morning, it will have a light coating. This is normal. A heavy or darker coloured coating indicates toxicity within the body. Some people use tongue-scrapers, or a toothbrush, when brushing their teeth. (If you need a tongue-scraper, it is time to detox!)

48hrs after commencing your detox/fast, the coating on the tongue becomes heavier, as the body cleans house and toxins circulate in the bloodstream. You will see, over the course of your fast, the coating becoming lighter. For those who are particularly toxic, this can take upward of 30 days.

The other indicator of when to stop is when you feel well again. While visible arthritis symptoms can disappear, in as little as 10 days, it may need longer to ensure disease is truly vanquished.

Buying Supplements

At the retreat we make our own herbal supplements, since imports are difficult to get through customs, expensive, and there is no better supplement than that which nature provides, fresh, in your garden.

If you are not sure, one of the first places to start is your local health store. Beware corporate brands. You can also purchase what you need from Dr Schulze' online, herbal pharmacy. Or Dr Robert Morse Herbal Health Club.

"All disease is caused by some sort of blockage. Whether it's blocked blood, lymph, oxygen, nutrition, nerve impulse, emotional energy, spiritual energy, or even what the Chinese, Japanese or Indians refer to as Chi, Ki, or Prana. When an area of the body gets blocked, it gets sick. It's that simple."
- Dr. Richard Schulze

Chapter 30
Psychiatry – A Dark Art

Psychiatry is a book in itself. Language used in medicine, is also a book in itself. Take the word 'sedative' or 'sedate'. It's a nice word. Comforting, soothing, positive, appealing. Your mind is out of control, filled with dark, oppressive thoughts, exercising a form of tyranny upon you, so you cannot sleep, cannot function, can no longer relate to others. A living hell. The psychiatrist says "Don't worry, here is a sedative to calm you and help you sleep". It sounds as innocuous as a mug of Horlicks or Ovaltine. Who wouldn't be seduced? Yet, what if the psychiatrist said,

"Here is a poison which will make you docile, destroy your sexual function, cause permanent brain changes and turn you into a life-long addict. And, by the way, it causes the very symptoms you are trying to relieve, will give you diabetes, trigger violent or suicidal thoughts and block you from reaching higher states of consciousness".

Still have that warm, fuzzy feeling?

Psychiatry wraps itself in medical clothes but lacks any credible science. An ever-increasing list of normal human behaviours is voted a 'disorder', with a show of hands, by members of the **American Psychiatric Association**, most of whom have ties to pharmaceutical companies. The result? The mass poisoning of society with fluorides and opiates.

'Drug companies allegedly paid seven figures to three Harvard professors of psychiatry -- Joseph Biederman, Thomas Spencer, and Timothy Wilens -- who then went on to encourage diagnosing children with bipolar disorder and medicating them with antipsychotic drugs.' - **Dr. Peter Breggin**

The 'Bible' of Psychiatry is called the **"Diagnostic and Statistical Manual"** (DSM). The latest version, DSM-5, is basically a billing system for insurance companies and governments.

Psychiatry is not a science. It's a Dark Art. Appropriate for a few seriously disturbed individuals, not the wholesale drugging of the masses.

Psychiatry has a history that is medieval in its barbarity and cruelty. While some of the more gruesome practices have ended, running electricity through someone's body and administering fluoride-based 'chemical coshes', to adults and infants alike, is inflicting State-sponsored violence upon the individual. Hippocrates instruction to 'first do no harm' is nowhere to be found.

1 in 4 adult Americans have been diagnosed with a mental disorder in the last 12 months. Diagnoses include major depression, bipolar disorder, schizophrenia and anxiety disorders, eating disorders, attention deficit disorder/attention deficit hyperactivity disorder (ADD/ADHD) and addiction. Worldwide, incidence rates range from a staggering 26% of the population in America, to 4% in China. That statistic, alone, should tell you something is seriously amiss in America.

What is behind this incredible rise? Are there really so many 'Mad Dads' (as someone once labelled me) 'Crazy Mums' and 'Barmy Kids' out there? Of course not. Most psychiatric disorders are inventions. Disease-mongers have created the illusion of widespread mental illness. The normal vagaries of life, labelled a 'disorder', for corporate profit and population control. When 2-year olds are diagnosed with 'Bipolar Disorder' and drugged, you are not looking at medicine but evil. Billions of dollars can be made from the sale of one drug... even a bad drug... if you have the right marketing campaign. Psychiatric drugs generate $billions.

Alternative medicine is castigated and dismissed for 'not having any science to support it', yet Psychiatry has less and is fully supported by government. Where is the test for a chemical imbalance of the brain? I have never seen or been offered one. Yet the industry still rides this unproven myth. The psychiatric equivalent of, "It's genetic".

Emotional trauma can be upsetting and some people need support. This used to be provided by extended family, community and the local priest. The vast majority of mental health problems are due to nutritional deficiency, poverty, poor parenting, war, toxic environment, lack of education, and the mass media pouring negativity, conflict and fear into our minds. Stress is a major cause of physical and mental illness.

The term 'Toxic Stress' has been coined to describe it. This Harvard article (17) explains:

'When toxic stress response occurs continually, or is triggered by multiple sources, it can have a cumulative toll on an individual's physical and mental health—for a lifetime. The more adverse experiences in childhood, the greater the likelihood of developmental delays and later health problems, including heart disease, diabetes, substance abuse, and depression.'

If I am experiencing stress because I have lost my job or am going through a painful divorce, or because the media are instilling fear in me, the way to relieve that stress is to provide me with employment, repair the relationship and switch off the TV. Poisoning my body and brain does nothing to resolve the underlying cause. A disturbed child does not need fluoride, or Class II narcotics, like Ritalin. He or she needs a secure, safe, supportive environment.

Young brains ARE subjected to an increasing number of developmental toxins, such as glutamine, aspartame, fluoride, lead, arsenic, pcb's, toluene, vaccine ingredients and more. The young are turned into uncontrollable monsters via subversive messages in cartoons and on TV. They are trained to defy parents and demand ice cream, burgers, coke and sweets. Teens are turned into sexualized sluts and knuckle-dragging thugs, by a corrupt music industry, whose intent is the degradation of society. It certainly isn't to elevate it. Is the remedy for this really to imbibe more poison?

Once again, you see that none of this is accidental. A drug-peddling Psychiatric industry being fed a steady supply of burned-out, confused and stressed customers.

The steady diet of 'zombie' movies from Hollywood is a perverse celebration of man being separated from the Divine. Millions are kept trapped in a waking sleep, their senses stupefied. No highs, no lows. You function but are dead to any feeling. Try to end dependence on chemicals and your anxiety worsens and suicidal thoughts arise. The name 'Hollywood' is interesting. Did you know the ancient English druids cast spells using a 'magic wand'? The wand was made from the wood of the holly tree. Holly... wood... Hollywood. Hollywood is a 'caster of spells'. Not only Hollywood. The music industry, TV, Newspapers and the internet (awash with porn), are busy little bees, relentlessly working in lock-step, capturing our minds. Are these 'spell-binders' promoting peace of mind, love, compassion, tolerance, forgiveness, selflessness, harmony, social cohesion, happiness and cultural respect? Or are they promoting fear, terror, violence, selfishness, materialism, hatred for each other, warmongering, social engineering, instant gratification, 'anything goes'? Is this REALLY what you want to be feeding your mind and the minds of your children? Think about it.

It has been my observation many Psychiatrists are themselves troubled. They chose this career path to work out their own inner demons and haven't managed it. If they cannot fix themselves, how can they fix their patients?

Drug-peddling works. The pharmaceutical industry makes staggering amounts of money, mountains of it. The medical and psychiatric professions make money. Their political partners-in-crime make money. Insurers make money. The loser is the patient who ends up a 'Zombie'. Peter Gotzsche, Danish physician, medical researcher and leader of the **Nordic Cochrane Center** has described the largest pharmaceutical companies as fitting the description of organized crime. It is hard to disagree.

When it comes to cleaning your mind, you might wish to start with all the implanted psychological and spiritual poison you have absorbed throughout a lifetime. Apply the **First Law of Healing**. Whatever you are doing that is making you sick, STOP DOING IT. Turn OFF your TV, STOP watching Hollywood movies and cartoons. STAY AWAY from pornography sites. Don't allow the 'casters of spells' to capture and poison your mind. Then apply **The Second Law**. Feed your mind the positive qualities I listed.

'I will follow that system of regimen which, according to my ability and judgment, I consider for the benefit of my patients, and abstain from whatever is deleterious and mischievous. I will give no deadly medicine to anyone if asked, nor suggest any such counsel.'
- Extract of the Hippocratic Oath

Stress-Related Disorders

We live in a highly stressful world. The effect on our nervous systems and psyche, of prolonged stress, is significant and cumulative. Millions lack peace of mind, triggering a cascade of physical disorders and addictions. Those that aren't self-tranquillizing are on a cocktail of psychiatric drugs. The mass drugging of children is a scandal and tragedy.

Thoughts and emotions powerfully affect brain, endocrine and immune system function. When we are stressed, specific hormones are secreted which allow us to run faster or fight harder. However, if sustained for longer periods of time, or unused, they inhibit the immune system. Chronic stress triggers physical and psychological disorders and exacerbates existing ones. In a 2010 study, researchers in the Netherlands proved that high levels of cortisol, a stress hormone, damage the cardiovascular system.

What other disorders does stress influence? Almost anything you can think of. Asthma, diabetes, obesity, depression and anxiety, heartburn, IBS, arthritis, accelerated aging and premature death. Stress produces tension in mind and body, via the 'Fight or Flight' response. When we are angry or fearful, our breathing becomes shallow. Thinking is 'foggy', concentration poor and short-term memory impaired. Cortisol blocks the creation of new synapses in the brain, preventing learning. Under stress, making even simple choices can initiate a crisis. Prolonged tension leads to high blood pressure, restricted blood, lymph and nerve flow and impaired digestion. Tension also upsets our acid/alkali balance. If you test the ph of your saliva, when under stress, you will find it more acidic. Dis-stress creates uncomfortable thoughts and feelings, so we turn up the volume on the radio, or reach for alcohol, food, sex, gambling and drugs. We 'self-harm'. These activities, while providing distraction, have negative consequences. Alcoholism, obesity, financial loss and addiction.

Stress Curve

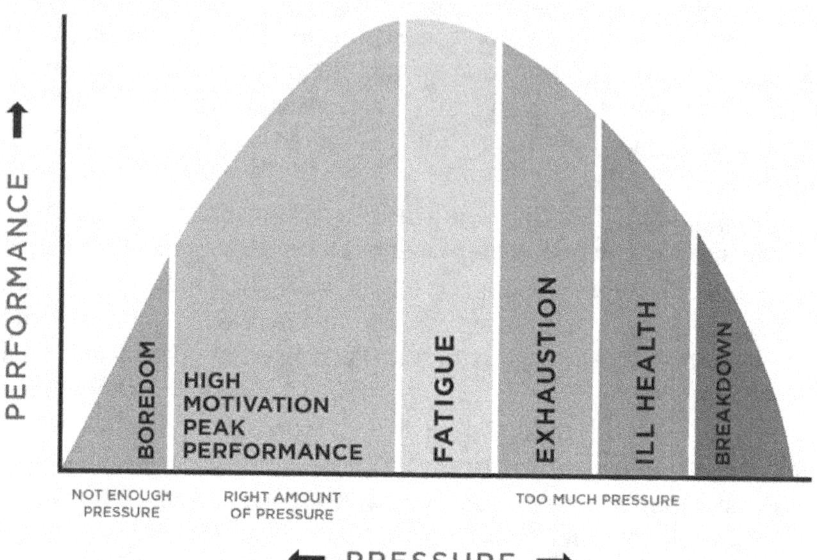

The chart shows the relationship between stress and performance. Some stress is good for us, improving performance. As pressure increases, we move from boredom to breakdown.

Where are you on the curve? MOst of us are somewhere between fatigue and breakdown.

What Do We Know About Stress?

- It is cumulative.
- Most of us are unaware of how tense we are.
- If stress is not resolved, we will be forced to resolve it.
- A minor event can tip people over the edge.
- Burying one's head in the sand does not solve problems.
- If you think you are 'mad', or 'going mad', you are not. Your body and mind are reacting to stress exactly as they should. You need education more than medication.
- Relationships do not break down when life is going well but under pressure. If a relationship does not have a strong foundation, it can collapse. How are your foundations?

Sources of Stress

Physical

- Chemical and heavy metal poisoning via food, air, water, vaccines and pharmaceuticals.
- Bacteria, virus, fungi and parasites
- Energetic imbalances: electrical cables, cell phone transmitters, computers, mobile phones.
- Congestion and stagnation of lymph, arteries, skin, liver, kidneys, nerve channels and bowel, leading to the accumulation of toxins and metabolic wastes. Constipation and lack of activity increase stress.
- Radiation via irradiated food, medical devices, airport scanners, x-rays, nuclear power plants and depleted uranium used in munitions.

Psychological

- Toxic emotions and thoughts. Fear, anxiety, anger leading to physical and psychological tension. These can include 'spiritual' blockages.
- Relationships, with people being divided and set against each other. Feminism, homosexuality, political correctness and attacks against Religion. Schools are 'dumbed down'. Politics is a circus, dominated by professional liars. The media swamp us with sensation, propaganda, 'dark' programming, fear, base language and immorality.
- Poverty is a major cause of stress and illness. Poor quality housing, inner city violence and crime, financial insecurity, unemployment, homelessness, drugs.

Nutritional Deficiency

- Medical conditions such as Crohn's, ulcerative colitis, Celiac disease or persistent diarrhoea, causing malabsorption.
- Eating disorders, such as anorexia or bulimia.
- Medicines which disrupt the body's ability to absorb and break down nutrients
- Failing to take proper care of oneself, such as drug addicts and alcoholics.
- Eating food deficient in essential vitamins and minerals.

- You may have a physical disability or other impairment that makes it difficult for you to cook, or shop for food, yourself. Limited knowledge of preserving nutrients during cooking.
- Incorrect diet for your Constitutional type.
- Undereating. Common in the elderly

In industrial societies millions are fat yet malnourished. In Asia, where food is an important part of the social fabric, they are catching up fast. 1 billion people around the world are classed as clinically obese. In the UK, the most common causes of malnutrition in children are long-term health conditions that either:

• Cause low appetite
• Disrupt the normal process of digestion
• Cause the body to have an increased demand for energy

Examples include childhood cancers, congenital heart disease, cystic fibrosis and cerebral palsy.

Life Stress Test

Stress is cumulative. The following is a list of stressful events with a score against it. To measure risk of illness, select all events occurring in the past year, then add up the total. Your final score gives an estimate of whether you will become ill.

1. Death of a spouse 100
2. Divorce 73
3. Marital separation 65
4. Imprisonment 63
5. Death of a close family member 63
6. Personal injury or illness 53
7. Marriage 50
8. Dismissal from work 47
9. Marital reconciliation 45
10. Retirement 45
11. Change in health of family member 44
12. Pregnancy 40
13. Sexual difficulties 39
14. Gain a new family member 39
15. Business readjustment 39
16. Change in financial state 38
17. Death of a close friend 37
18. Change to different line of work 36

19. Change in frequency of arguments 35
20. Major mortgage 32
21. Foreclosure of mortgage or loan 30
22. Change in responsibilities at work 29
23. Child leaving home 29
24. Trouble with in-laws 29
25. Outstanding personal achievement 28
26. Spouse starts or stops work 26
27. Beginning or end school 26
28. Change in living conditions 25
29. Revision of personal habits 24
30. Trouble with boss 23
31. Change in working hours or conditions 20
32. Change in residence 20
33. Change in schools 20
34. Change in recreation 19
35. Change in church activities 19
36. Change in social activities 18
37. Minor mortgage or loan 17
38. Change in sleeping habits 16
39. Change in number of family reunions 15
40. Change in eating habits 15
41. Vacation 13
42. Major Holiday 12
43. Minor violation of law 11

Score of 300+: High risk of illness.
Score of 150-299: Moderate risk of illness
Score <150: Slight risk of illness.

Taken from "The Social Readjustment Rating Scale", Thomas H. Holmes and Richard H. Rahe, **Journal of Psychosomatic Research**, Volume 11, Issue 2, August 1967

Controlling a Troubled Mind

The list of stressors is varied and lengthy, involving dietary, environmental and social factors. The idea you can take a single supplement and stress and illness will evaporate is unlikely. To be healthy and happy, we need to look at every aspect of our lives, how we manage stress and how we nourish our bodies and minds.

Where you are unable to change something, like environment, all is not lost. One of the most iconic symbols in Asia is the Lotus Flower, which grows in muddy water, yet produces wonderful blossoms. Like the Lotus, we can thrive, despite adverse circumstances.

When well balanced, our minds are calm, clear-thinking and a useful tool. When out of balance they become tyrannical. Fearful thoughts, angry thoughts, useless thoughts, sexual thoughts, dark and repetitive thoughts. Constantly swirling around in our mental soup. We feel powerless to calm the mind because we have been trained to look outward for solutions, never inward. We do not believe we can control or change our thoughts. Most of the time, we are not even aware of what we are thinking. On both the Online Health Coaching programs and Retreats we teach how to change thinking so that, like the Lotus flower, you can blossom in a challenging environment.

Most people wander around, on automatic-pilot, in a kind of dream-like state. Eating, walking, driving, talking. With no real idea of what they are thinking. Neither aware, nor in the present moment. Instead minds are preoccupied with the past or future, (when not glued to a smartphone). Like computers, we have an input and output. What we output reflects what is input. So we program… or allow others to program… our minds with all kinds of beliefs and ideas. When we are sat, unconsciously munching, in front of TV or movie screen, there is very little filtering of what goes into our minds.

As mentioned previously, we are constantly being told what to think, what to believe, what to eat, what to wear, who to like, who to hate, who is in and who is out. Passive acceptance of these messages is dangerous to psychological health. The mind needs to be nourished with positive, powerful, loving messages. Yet what is fed us by mainstream media? Hate, sensationalism, division, propaganda, immorality and 200 channels of stupefying rubbish.

'Garbage in, Garbage out'.

Not only does media brainwashing shape our beliefs, it over-stimulates the nervous system. The rapidly changing images and roller-coaster of fear, excitement and anger, exhaust our adrenals and destroy our concentration until we end up unable to relax, and addicted to each new stimuli. We eventually become bored, needing ever-increasing sensation to capture and hold our attention. A good place, therefore, to start reducing stress, is to ditch the media. I am far happier today, not reading newspapers, watching TV, Hollywood movies, or music videos. While the internet is undoubtedly addictive, YOU decide what you put into your mind, rather than accept what SOMEONE ELSE wants to feed you. It provides alternative viewpoints the mainstream media do not, or will not, present. Although that is rapidly changing. Everything we do online is tracked, so we become reluctant to honestly express our opinions. Alternative views are being side-lined, un-indexed or removed.

Take care with your internet use. There is a price to be paid for over-doing it. The repetitive 'clack-clack-clackety-clack' of fingers on keyboards, irritates our nervous system. Addiction, electro-magnetic radiation, lack of exercise, eyestrain and poor posture also create stress.

If your mind is full to overflowing, or thinking feels like you are ploughing through a muddy field, follow the advice of Air Force fighter pilots. They have 3 steps to staying focussed.

1. **Checklists**. Write down what you need to know.

2. **Cross-checking**. If you have a long list of tasks, take the top 5 most important tasks and double-check they are completed.

3. **Mutual support**. Have a friend, work colleague, buddy or family member back you up and spot anything you may miss.

"Many who are self-taught far excel the doctors, masters, and bachelors of the most renowned universities."
- Ludwig von Mises

Chapter 31
Who Am I?

I am an ordinary man, with a passion for truth and compassion for others. A career in the military and love of travel have seen me spend much of my life travelling and living abroad. Today, I am settled, although kept busy with retreats, online health coaching and writing books like this. Health-wise, I learned 'auto-didactically'… meaning I am mostly self-taught… with twenty five years investigating natural methods of healing to find a cure for my own chronic disorders.

I am not an academic, professional author or licenced medical practitioner. I provide education and support to those in need, writing as a consumer and natural healing advocate. Health fascinates me and there is always more to learn. During the last two and a half decades I have become versed in numerous healing techniques, both their theory and practical application. The Thomsonian School of Healing, Gandhi's 'Nature Cure', Ayurveda and more. The latter two I studied in Kerala, India, the 'Home of Ayurveda'. I teach Yoga as therapy, along with several meditation techniques, can design nutritional healing plans, and give a passable Thai Massage. 2 years in a Raja Yoga Retreat taught me much about stress and mastery over the mind. EFT+NLP, 'Breaking The Chains', juice and water fasting, Reiki, oxygen therapies and herbalism were all added to my Holistic Healing Toolkit.

Living several years next to a healing retreat, where visiting practitioners would hold regular workshops, considerably expanded my knowledge. As did a long period of experimentation with esoteric-minded friends, learning about local herbs and how to prepare them. We practiced breathing exercises, bodywork, hydrotherapy, organic gardening, psychological and emotional healing. Pretty much the whole gamut of natural therapies.

With every new technique I encountered, I kept an open mind and did not allow anyone else to decide for me who was a charlatan and what was 'quackery' (the Health Industry's code word for 'competition'). This was a world apart from my previous attitude, with absolute faith and acceptance of modern medicine because it has been 'scientifically proven' and everything unproven was, therefore, bogus. A little investigation soon shattered that myth.

Today, whenever the corporate media run hit-pieces, going after alternative practices or practitioners (the competition), I no longer nod in approval, or snarl on command, but become intensely interested. "Why are they working so hard to demonize this person, supplement or technique? This is something I want to investigate". It is surprising what you learn.

On the psycho/emotional side my lengthy struggle with chronic anxiety, panic disorder and 'burn-out', gave me valuable insights into how ineffective psychiatry is and how depression, anger, anxiety and addictions can be resolved without resorting to harmful chemistry, or taking an electric drill to the side of my skull. Sceptics demand to know my medical qualifications, as if only the qualified have the right to comment on health matters. This is silliness. For most people, recovering health is very simple because the causes of their disorders are simple. If you believe in true freedom, as opposed to medical dictatorship, everyone has a right, even a moral imperative, to take care of themselves and others.

I am sometimes asked, *"You know so much about health. Why not qualify?"* In what? In conventional medicine the qualified are unable to cure chronic disease. They excel in **avoiding** cures and memorizing drug names. Of what use are such qualifications, to me?

According to the literature, around 100 years ago, allopathic medical education was taken over by the Rockefeller, Carnegie Corporations and JP Morgan bank, who skewed education toward pharmaceutical medicines, derived from crude oil. Improvement was certainly needed at the time. The profession endured a poor reputation. Medical Degrees could be easily purchased through the mail, or obtained with the minimum of training. Today, Doctors' medical education is high quality and their expertise praiseworthy. In disease management and pharmaceutical medicine, they excel. In emergency and acute disorders, they excel. Unfortunately, in nutrition, prevention, treating the whole person, addressing underlying cause and using non-toxic, non-invasive methods of healing, they are all at sea with their genomes and minimalist specializations.

It is hardly the Doctor's fault if their healing knowledge is non-existent. Their beliefs have been shaped by Corporations toward profitable treatments. They are highly qualified in '**Looking in the Wrong Direction**', ex-President Obama's '**Precision Medicine Initiative**', an example.

Here is my message to policy-makers. Forget genetics. Get out in the street and deal with the real killers in our midst. Poverty, violence, poor quality education, lack of opportunity, junk food, polluted relationships, toxic environment, corrupt media and politics, endless wars, social deprivation, and injustice.

Of what use is a qualification if not backed by ethical behaviour? Judging by the number of fines and prosecutions, of Doctors, in recent years, the Health Industry has abandoned ethics. 95% of Doctors in America have taken 'inducements' from drug companies – free meals, tickets to the basketball game, seminars in the Bahamas or Cancun – to encourage them to prescribe the latest 'blockbuster' drug, rather than cheaper, more effective medicines, whose patents have expired. Lead Doctors are shamelessly on the drug companies' payroll.

What about Alternative Medicine Schools? **Bastyr University,** in the U.S., has an interesting **Ayurvedic Master of Science** program, covering medical Sanskrit, psychology, yoga, pathology, herbal therapies and nutrition. I've been studying Ayurveda since before it became fashionable. A Doctor of Naturopathy is another possibility but I am getting a bit long in the tooth to go back to school.

Ethical questions surround alternative practitioners, too. Many have entered the health field to do one thing and one thing only. Make money. An army of practitioners have qualified, via Correspondence Course, or night school, in minor therapies like massage, Reiki, EFT and so on. This allows them to make a living. However, ask them where the gall bladder or spleen is and they have no idea. They know nothing of Anatomy and Physiology. It may not be necessary for them to know but you can understand why conventional medicine is dismissive. How can someone doing a 2-day Reiki course compare to a Doctor who has spent 12 years in high-level study?

Why is it NOT necessary for Alternative practitioners to learn Anatomy and Physiology? Well, their particular discipline may not require it. Do I need to know the inner workings of my car's engine to give it the right fuel?

Doctors' lack of ethics and insufferable arrogance is damning. They have the gall to dismiss anything natural that might help patients. Their arrogance is summed up nicely in this poem from the late 1800's:

> *'Tis nature that does it – but what right has she*
> *To be round curing people without a degree?*
> *A man to be cured without sending for me!*
> *Without sending for any right licenced M.D.!!*
> *It's unscientific, irregular, mean----*
> *The shamefulest thing that ever was seen!'*

'Mad Dads' and 'Crazy Mums'

25 years ago, after a sustained period of stress, I broke down. Physically, psychologically, emotionally and spiritually. Ten years later I came within a whisker of breaking down again. I was 'burnt-out', suffering chronic anxiety, panic attacks and living in a 'dark pit of despair' (if you have ever been 'in the pit', you will understand).

What could have upset my mind to the extent I needed to spend 3 ½ years on anti-depressants, just to sleep? The possibilities seem endless. I spent a decade trying to understand what happened to me and why I was unable to bounce back. Having seen Doctors, Psychiatrists and therapists of every stripe, I began to build a picture. Each interaction, another brick in my wall of understanding. 20 different psychiatrists would give me 20 different reasons why I was depressed and anxious, all of which sounded plausible. The solution, though, always came back to chemistry. The need to correct some 'chemical imbalance in the brain', for which no test exists. I didn't understand then, but certainly do now, the poisons they gave me, were not **correcting** imbalances but **creating** them.

Delving into a troubled mind is like falling down the rabbit-hole in **Alice in Wonderland**. You enter a chaotic landscape, filled with imaginary creatures that seem all too real. After following umpteen different trails, I was completely lost. Was I really sexually abused as a child? Was some dark family secret, from generations ago, pervading my present psyche? Did my inner child need a hug? Was my previously dormant soul awakening? My self-esteem or self-confidence, too low? Was it Social Anxiety Disorder? Post-Traumatic Stress Disorder? Generalized Anxiety Disorder? Gulf War Syndrome? Mercury or radiation-poisoning? Adrenal Exhaustion? Anti-depressants, **causing** the very anxiety and suicidal thoughts they claim to relieve? (Interesting how many drugs do this).

I was dead to all feeling, doped with Seroxat, an SSRI class of psychiatric drug, containing Fluoride. Other brand names are:

Citalopram (Celexa)

Escitalopram (Lexapro)

Fluoxetine (Prozac)

Paroxetine (Paxil, Pexeva)

Sertraline (Zoloft)

If fluoride can have such a numbing effect on my brain I can understand the controversy over dumping millions of tons of it into our water supply, adding it to toothpaste and an increasing number of products. That aside, I was initially grateful for the extra sleep it afforded me. Until the side effects began to manifest, which the Doctor somehow forgot to mention as he wrote his prescription. Addiction, permanent brain changes, chronic fatigue, suicidal thoughts and sexual dysfunction. My once-vital sex life deteriorated and has been… ahem… up and down ever since.

"Thanks, Doc."

After years of getting nowhere, I finally wrapped all the theories up in a large black bag labelled 'psychobabble' and tossed them in the bin. Later, I came to a startling realization. It was NONE of those things. All these suspected causes disappeared in a puff of smoke once I identified and corrected the **physical** cause. The specialist in Bangkok had been right all along. I had **Celiac Disease**. This disorder had wiped out all the microvilli in my intestines (these microscopic hairs absorb nutrients from food). Modern diets are already nutritionally deficient. For me, the problem was compounded because I was unable to extract nutrients, even if they were present. Support for Hippocrates who said,

"All disease begins in the gut".

A common symptom of Celiac Disease is depression and anxiety, since the brain is starved of nutrients. Symptoms manifest as being 'all in the mind', so we are referred to psychiatry, which is armed and ready to club the mind into submission with an array of poisons. Of all the experts I saw over the years, psychiatrists, psychotherapists, hypnotherapists, etc.., not one considered there may be a **physical** cause to my psychological problems. Not one realized vital nutrients, which provide resilience to stress, had been gobbled up by life events, until my nutrient bank was empty. I was not deficient in Prozac or Valium or Beta-blockers or Seroxat but B1, B2, B3, B5, B12, Folic Acid, fats and oils. My adrenal glands (produce stress hormones) were worn out from spending too many years in 'fight or fight' mode. I was not so much a 'Mad Dad' but a **starving** dad. Nor was I alone. 18 million adults in the U.S. suffer anxiety disorders. 350 million people around the world suffer depression, more women than men. Could it be that, for many of these millions, the root of their problem lies not on the psychiatrist's couch but on the dinner table?

'Nutritional Neuroscience' is starting to shed light on this (18):

'…essential vitamins, minerals, and omega-3 fatty acids are often deficient in the general population in America and other developed countries; and are exceptionally deficient in patients suffering from

mental disorders. Studies have shown that daily supplements of vital nutrients often effectively reduce patients' symptoms.'

Oh yes. Must not forget. Remember the Naturopath who said he could have cured me in 3 days? His remedy? Niacin. Up to 8mg per day. **Orthomolecular Medicine**, means healing through nutrition. Advocates, like the insightful Andrew Saul, provide numerous examples of Niacin working wonders on psychiatric patients. This would not have resolved the Celiac Disease (the gut villi needed to be restored) but it may very well have relieved my anxiety and panic attacks, without the need for drugs.

Chronic stress and its effects on our health are a recognized problem. In warfare, 30% of servicemen consistently experience some kind of stress disorder. If I could study them, I am sure most would be Ayurvedic 'Air' Types (see Addendum for a description). This Constitutional Type tend toward nervous disorders. Ayurveda identified them, thousands of years ago.

Chronic stress can seriously threaten physical and emotional well-being, triggering psychosomatic illness. There exists a huge lack of understanding of what stress is, its causes, how pressure builds up over time and how it can be dealt with, effectively, at an early stage.

Having taken the decision to escape the pressure I was under (an action I should have taken a decade before), I set about restoring my psychological and physical health. My joints were painful, there were seasonal allergies and, over the years, heart disease (chest pain), fibromyalgia, inflammatory bowel disease, hypoglycaemia, enlarged prostate and inguinal hernias. My hands trembled, I bruised easily, was constantly fatigued and underweight. Tension headaches, foggy thinking, poor concentration and memory were the norm.

The physical ailments were almost all due to prolonged tension. Tension in the mind causes tension in the body and vice-versa. When muscles and tendons are tight, blood flow, nerve flow, lymph flow and vital energy are restricted or blocked. The constant circulation of stress hormones upsets the digestive system, along with the acid/alkaline balance. Stress affects the **whole** person.

Chemicals. Antibiotics. Painkillers. Anti-inflammatories. Anti-histamines. Beta-blockers. Anti-anxiety medication. Muscle-relaxants. Chemical after chemical were prescribed. After years of this, I understood. No Doctor or psychiatrist was going to CURE me. How could they? They had no idea what was wrong with me.'

I realized I would have to cure myself.

Abandoning Ship

After 'The Peace That Passeth All Understanding' had ebbed away, my stress returned, my marriage started to fail and I was back on Seroxat, heading for that second nervous breakdown. With my joints increasingly painful, I had no choice in the matter. In my anxiety-filled state, visions of an early grave, if I did not act, appalled me. I had to get away.

The unsympathetic portrayed my need to escape and recover as 'running away'. Evidence of a lack of moral character. They believe we all have crises at some point in our lives and should simply shrug them off, pick ourselves up and carry on. As if this wasn't blindingly obvious and I hadn't struggled for years to do precisely that. Of course, I and my loved ones wished all had been well. Had the events that tipped me into crisis not taken place, my life and the lives of those around me might have been very different. Yet, it was not to be. Whatever the effect on others of my leaving, I was of no use to anyone as a suicide statistic.

Now, you may not have the time, money, or opportunity to retreat into the wilderness. BUT if you are suicidal or dying from disease, you must do whatever it takes to get well.

I jumped on a motorbike, left everything behind, crossed the English Channel, rode over the Alps, travelled down through the Pyrenees, into Portugal, where I landed on a barren hillside in the Algarve. After a year of isolation in a derelict farmhouse, exercising my body, with Hatha Yoga, I spent 2 years in a Raja Yoga retreat, learning how the mind works and techniques for bringing it under control. No need for me to remain at the mercy of my mind any longer. I could become its Master!

The flavour of Raja Yoga I embraced, encouraged purity. Purity of thought, purity of action, pure food, celibacy and knowledge of how to live one's life. Combined with meditation, I experienced a noticeable improvement. Observers would remark on how brilliant and clear my eyes were (the 'Windows to the Soul'). My body certainly felt clean. Yet, for all its benefits, recovery wasn't complete. I was 80% better. Good but not good enough.

Living a life of celibacy was easy after the initial trauma of separation and divorce. The last thing I wanted, during this period, was another relationship. But as time passed and my vitality and optimism returned, so did the twinkle in my eye. Repressing one's natural urges isn't wise, as many an unfrocked Priest has discovered. The sexual urge is one of the strongest instincts in man. While I could have spent the rest of my life as an ascetic, possibly happier in a retreat than the 'normal' world, I knew it was time to leave.

Two years and more, of meditation, had shown me one thing. How difficult it was to settle the western mind. I observed this many times during group sessions. Western nervous systems are so over-stimulated we cannot sit still for five minutes. We have lost the ability to relax or concentrate. Many give up on meditation. Defeated by their bodies. This is why Hatha Yoga is an integral part of the Ayurvedic/Yoga system. The body needs to be trained to properly relax, and the mind to concentrate, BEFORE meditation is possible. If you find yourself fidgeting too much, don't be discouraged. Particularly 'Air Types, with their tendency to nervousness. Work on relaxation and concentration.

The Long Dark Night of the Soul

This period in my life was, without doubt, the most difficult I have ever had to endure. A lengthy and profound absence of light and hope. Breaking down. in a pit of despair. Profoundly alone. Suicide the only way out.

Imagine only getting one hour's sleep per night. The pressure in your head so intense you want to drill a hole in your temple to relieve it. Fear and anxiety so overwhelming your heart is constantly pounding. You feel like you cannot breathe, you are dying, or 'going crazy'. Imagine experiencing this for months. Today, if you were to ask me about this period, I would call it a blessing. The prelude to re-birth. A stage I had to go through to transform from the old to the new. Cancer survivors sometimes say their cancer was the best thing that ever happened to them because it forced them to re-evaluate and take a good look at themselves. To alter their disease-inducing lifestyles; re-examine their values and beliefs and emerge from their disease with an improved outlook on life. I am certainly not unique. 10% of people go through a major crisis at some point in their lives, asking profound questions:

"Who am I?"

"What is my purpose in life?"

"Is this all there is?"

Was I just an entry in a government and corporate database, branded and tracked, from birth, by my social security number? Estimated by corporate bean-counters to be worth $1,000,000 in future profits as soon as I exit the womb? A conditioned drone, living a pre-determined, material existence until death or taxes finish me. Surely my value as a human being was worth more than a pointless vote every four years to decide which set of white-collar criminals get to plunder the public purse? We are much more than this. Organized religion may have been discredited by its corrupt leaders and the decades-long campaign by the media to destroy it but I would rather be seen as a wonderful, unique, creation of 'God', a place reserved for me at his right hand, than a profit opportunity for the already wealthy.

Few of my military colleagues will live to collect their full pensions. I have heard the official figure is as low as 11%. My father, an ex-soldier, died the day his first pension cheque hit the bank. He was 55. My father-in-law, empty whisky bottle in his hand, died at 49. A lawyer friend, 50, died when his heart gave out. Life is precious and short. Though, yesterday, I may have suffered. Today, I am grateful to be alive.

Which leads me to make a plea. If you are ever faced with an individual who is stressed, or suicidal, try not to condemn them. You have no idea what they may have been through (particularly war veterans). They do not need your condemnation. Along with physical, emotional and psychological support, sufferers need patience, tolerance and understanding. They also require proper nutrition. Show a little compassion. Next time it could be you.

I Fired My Doctor!

My GP was compassionate but showed no interest in me beyond prescribing anti-depressants. Military psychiatric nurses commendably introduced me to non-drug approaches, like relaxation training and stress management, with little effect. Over time, it became clear. Firing my Doctor was the only realistic resort.

You can save a lot of time by asking your Doctor a simple question, *"CAN YOU CURE ME?"*

By that, I mean can your Doctor create the conditions which will allow your body and mind to heal? If the answer is "No", walk away. Unless you are content with relief of symptoms. Some people are.

After walking away, the first step was to find space and time to come off anti-depressants. I exchanged my comfortable home, in England, for a dilapidated farmhouse in the Algarve, with no running water and few amenities. Like something from a film set, my room was stark and empty, with white plaster falling off stone walls. A single bed, wooden chair and bare bulb provided only dim light. I showered, using cold water, from a bucket. There was nothing else. No TV. No radio. No computer. No phone. No ornamental clutter, requiring shelves and then more shelves, to accommodate it all. The perfect sanctuary for an ascetic monk and my wrecked nervous system.

The lack of visual and aural stimulation was exactly what was needed. Each day I would walk the lavender-covered hills, with not a soul to be seen. I could not run, my arthritic knees hurt. Yoga became my chosen exercise. For five hours a day I practiced. Three hours in the morning and two in the afternoon. I adopted a vegan diet, breathed in unpolluted air, sunbathed, read self-help books and learned as much as I could about mental and physical health. Eventually my efforts started to bear fruit. My nerves began to settle, mind began to calm and, despite an alarming 3 months (I failed the first time), coming off Seroxat, I started to feel somewhat human again.

I failed on my first attempt to come off the anti-depressants, after a frightening wave of anxiety and suicidal thinking hit me. No wonder so many are trapped on these drugs for life. It isn't just anxiety and suicide. Anger can increase on withdrawal. Ask the school shooters in America.

It had taken me a year to reach this stage. While I was over the worst, I wasn't cured. The winters in Portugal were a challenge. Properties were not built for cold weather and during weeks of rainfall, my arthritis flared. The vegan diet, supposedly the best diet for health, left me tired and undernourished and I was still carrying around a deep, unresolved fear I would end up like my mother.

What did my mother have to do with it? Plenty. All my mental and physical symptoms? My mother had experienced, before me, and she endured a painful and prolonged death. Scripture informs us the 'Sins of the fathers shall be visited upon the children'. Was my disease inherited? 'Bad blood' or weak semen? Had I been poisoned by chemicals in my mother's breast milk? What about HER mercury fillings, or vaccines? Could they have injured me in the womb? If so, why not my brother and sister?

You often see children develop the same disorders as their parents, simply because they are consuming the same disease-inducing diet. Were my mother and I sensitive to the same foods? There were indicators of food sensitivity from an early age. A runny nose after eating porridge (oatmeal). Mouth ulcers after eating biscuits or popcorn. When young, you pay little attention.

My mother struggled most of her adult life with illness. Some real. Some imagined. She embraced hypochondria like a warm blanket. Sickness kept my social father home and brought her attention. After years of feigning illness, we children were drained of any sympathy.

Eventually she developed full blown Rheumatoid Arthritis, the treatment of which eventually killed her. Her last two years of life were a torment, with constant pain and botched operations. She learned about medical 'complications' the hard way. After one trip to the Intensive Care Unit, due to a surgical error, she was left needing a colostomy bag for the rest of her days. You could feel her humiliation and sadness.

This was the future I was facing and it terrified me. Orthodox treatments for Rheumatoid Arthritis have barely changed. A painful and prolonged death. An overdose of morphine eventually put her out of her misery, giving weight to Moliere's words, uttered hundreds of years ago,

"Nearly all men die of their remedies and not of their illnesses."

Shopping at the Alternative Healing Bazaar

For many years after firing my Doctor, I immersed myself in the murky waters of alternative practitioners and their techniques. Acupuncture, Cranial Osteopathy, Chiropractic, Traditional Chinese Medicine, Ayurveda (both ancient and modern), Thai Traditional Medicine, Homeopaths, Osteopaths, Naturopaths, Astrologers, Faith Healers, Mediums, Reiki Masters, Herbalists, Yogis, Hypnotherapists, Shamen, Sufi and Christian priests. Emotional and spiritual healers. An endless number of 'Wonder Cures', available online, all major credit cards accepted.

I became educated in alternatives and could impress everyone with my knowledge. On my travels, I met others just like me, who had shopped at the Alternative Healing Bazaar. Highly knowledgeable, yet still not cured.

Then there are those who do not practice what they preach. I know an Ayurvedic Doctor who teaches Yoga and meditation and offers healthy Indian food. His stomach expands each time I see him.

If you are extolling the virtues of juice fasting and how wonderful it is for your skin, it doesn't help if your own looks like orange peel. If you are teaching how to balance the autonomic nervous system, it does not look good if you cannot sit still. If marketing weight loss products, it doesn't look good if you are overweight. Or, leading a spiritual life. Like the monks in certain parts of Asia, who smoke. If you are a psychiatrist, it doesn't help your credibility if you look like an axe-murderer. When I see practitioners who do not take care of themselves, Jesus instruction, *"Physician, heal thyself"* springs to mind.

My Introduction to Ayurveda

Ayurveda is far more than Hatha and Raja Yoga. It incorporates values and morals, nutrition, herbs, detoxification, as well as astrological components. It is a total holistic system.

In 2004, hearing good things about Ayurveda, I decided to investigate. So, it was off to Kerala, India, the 'Home of Ayurveda', with a friend who had Leukaemia. We found an authentic clinic where they set to work. For 44 consecutive days, I received a variety of treatments, twice daily, from both ancient and modern forms. Following that, I spent a month at a 'Nature Cure' Centre. Watching elephants logging, in the middle of the jungle, added to the sense of authenticity.

In both systems, only safe, natural methods are used, with not a bleeping, radiating machine in sight. The idea you can not only treat but cure patients, without technology, was something novel. My arthritis symptoms resolved and my circulation was restored. My hands and feet, normally cold, were as warm as toast. My rock-hard muscles were supple and relaxed. All tension in my body was gone. The cost was remarkably cheap.

After several months in India I left, inspired by what I had seen. I shall always be grateful to the humble, pot-bellied, Hindu 'Vaidya' (traditional Ayurvedic Doctor), constantly standing on one leg, muttering mantras and counting his Mala beads, who tended to me.

I had met my first authentic natural healer.

This curious man, who spoke no English, did more for me in a month with his massage and herbs than any 'scientific' Doctor ever did with their drugs. What struck me about the Vaidya, wasn't just the religious and cultural strangeness, which would cause most westerners to dismiss him. But the extent of his knowledge. I was shown a library of remedies, written on Papyrus, hundreds of years old, that had been passed down from generation to generation within his family.

So excited was I to have found Ayurveda and 'Nature Cure', I tried to share this new-found knowledge with a western-trained Doctor. I will never forget his disdainful dismissal. I have learned since, this closed-minded affliction, endemic amongst pharmaceutically-trained, western Doctors, is called, **'Doctor Brain'**.

"Worry and stress affect the circulation, the heart, the glands, the whole nervous system, and profoundly affects heart action"
- Charles W. Mayo, M.D

Chapter 32
Wisdom of the Ancients

India is not just synonymous with curries and population growth. It is considered the cradle of civilization. Much of our medical knowledge came from the ancient gurus and yogis of India. The ancients had a great understanding of the mind. They understood, thousands of years ago, what western Doctors and Psychiatrists fail to grasp. You cannot separate the head from the body and expect people to get better. So, it was to the ancients I turned when my body was hurting and my mind was in turmoil. In particular, the healing systems known as Ayurveda and Nature Cure.

Nature Cure

Naturopathy believes we fall ill when we violate the laws of nature, and all healing powers lie within the body. This is a different concept to that of mainstream medicine, particularly since the 1800's and the advent of 'heroic medicine'. This is when regular Doctors made Nature redundant and decided they could do a better (heroic) job of it. An example of this attitude is the teaching of medical professor Benjamin Rush, who advised students,

"Always treat nature in a sick room as you would a noisy dog or cat. Drive her out the door and lock it upon her".

Doctors' belief in the superiority of their methods has remained undiminished, even in the face of widespread failure, ever since. They may quote him but Hippocrates would disown the doctors of today. Hippocrates believed in nature, as did the founder of the Thomsonian School of Healing, Samuel Thomson. The fundamental 'vitalistic' principles of natural healing had not changed for a thousand years, when the 'Mechanists' decided to reduce the body to its physical and chemical constituents, rejecting 'Vitalism'.

Nature Cure is simple and based on common sense. Support the body's intrinsic efforts to heal. Use cleansing, diet, herbs, exercise, sunlight, hydrotherapy, stress reduction and (where people are open) spiritual power. In India I observed patients, rejected by hospitals and sent home to die, completely recover at Nature Cure Centres. Nature Cure might have been more widely taken up had it not been so simple.

Unfortunately, the public is more impressed by the complex and mysterious.

Ayurveda

What is Ayurveda? The name itself means 'Science of Life' or 'Knowledge of Life'. Its origins are said to go back 5000 years. The oldest system of lifestyle and medicine in the world. Ayurveda is a comprehensive, eco-friendly, holistic, 'Mind-Body' system of living that addresses the whole person. Ayurveda utilizes natural, non-toxic, non-invasive techniques to restore body, mind and spirit. These include the classic naturopathic components: nutrition, exercise, cleansing, bodywork, herbs, emotional healing and stress reduction.

In India, Ayurveda has two strands, ancient and modern, both of which are fully supported by the Indian Government and the World Health Organization. Two-thirds of India's rural people, 70% of the population, use Ayurveda for their primary health care needs. There are presently 400,000 Ayurvedic Doctors, who train as conventional medical Doctors, then go on to further qualify in Ayurveda and its sub-specializations.

Hatha Yoga

Yoga is a 'mind-body' system, designed to strengthen and relax the body. The ancients did not want a restless body interfering with meditation *(you cannot meditate if you cannot sit still)*. There are typically 3 parts. Asanas (physical exercises), Pranayama (breathing) and relaxation exercises. There are many schools of Yoga, such as Iyengar, Sivananda, Kundalini, Ashtanga and more. While only a minor part of the overall Ayurvedic system, Hatha Yoga is suitable for everyone, takes up little space, does not require equipment and once you grasp the basic moves, you can practice at home, at no cost. No need to pound pavements and stress those weight-bearing joints. Hatha Yoga relaxes the body, which calms the mind. A super introduction to Yoga is to find a '**Laughter Yoga**' class. It is not pure Yoga but is great fun all the same. 'Laughter is the BEST medicine!'

In the west, Hatha Yoga is treated as a physical exercise program rather than a method of improving self-awareness and achieving union. If you have practiced Yoga for any length of time, you understand how beneficial it is in strengthening and relaxing the body. Qi Gong and Tai Chi are similar 'mind-body' systems.

Raja Yoga

Raja Yoga means the 'Royal Path'. Raja Yoga focuses on mastery over the mind. It has techniques for controlling desires, improving concentration, bringing us back to our true nature and enjoying absolute peace and contentment. Raja Yoga sees no need for rigid physical postures, believing the mind will relax the body. In the Brahma Kumaris version of Raja Yoga, we sat on a comfy chair, or sofa, to meditate. 'Brahma Kumaris', a world-wide organization, affiliated to the United Nations, offers 'Positive Thinking' and 'Stress Management' courses for individuals and corporations, using Raja Yoga techniques. If you can find a branch near you, I highly recommend attending a class. Some people regard this organization as cult-like, so beware.

Raja Yoga and Hatha Yoga. The mind affects the body and the body affects the mind. One works from the outside-in. The other from the inside-out. You see? You can practice them separately but, in my experience, will achieve better results practicing them together.

Ice-Cream for the Mind

Transcendental Meditation (TM), introduced to the West, from India, in the late 50s, involves the repetition of one word, a mantra, which you practice for 10-20 minutes, twice a day. It is impossible to quiet an unruly mind by trying NOT to think. Struggle is force and you will find the mind becomes more agitated if you attempt to subdue it. The opposite of what you are seeking. The ancients learned, mechanically repeating a word (mantra), or phrase, has a settling effect on the mind. If you practice correctly, there is no effort. No struggle. The cost of a TM program can be high. However, when you give techniques away free, people tend not to apply them. High prices motivate people to practice, so as not to waste their money.

TM mantras are universal knowledge and should be accessible to all, not just those who can afford it, which is why I offer them to my retreat guests. The mantras are neither new nor unique. They are well known to Ayurveda. Just not in the West. There are subtle differences between mantras. You need to select (or be given) the mantra to suit your need, Chakra and constitutional type.

[In Yoga, chakras are energy centres that run from the top of the head to the base of the spine].

Chapter 33
Support is Critical

Do your loved ones want you to be well? This seems a bizarre question. Of course they do. But do they? While alternative therapies are becoming more widely accepted, anyone with a serious illness, who decides to **Fire Their Doctor** and try alternatives, can find themselves subjected to intense pressure from friends and family. To disregard 'unproven' methods and follow the officially prescribed route. Cancer, in particular. Unfortunately, while many are sincere, and think they know, they lack sufficient knowledge to be offering advice.

One reason people return to unhealthy patterns is because the husband, boyfriend, or significant other, objects. They do not want to eat 'rabbit food' (vegan or vegetarian diet), believe you are wasting your (or their) money. Or, deep down, fear you may change. Their instincts are correct. When you embark on a healing journey, more than just your diet has to change. You are addressing the whole person. Your beliefs, values, lifestyle and relationships... which may be toxic and a major cause of your illness... need to be examined. Healing from chronic disease can be simple and quick, or it can require major transformation. Such change can be frightening to those around you. They will fight to maintain things as they are, to keep you dependent on them. At first, supporting you, then undermining your efforts. Keeping at you until you surrender and give them the 'old' you they are comfortable with. Is this someone you know? Find out. Then ask yourself what is more important? Your health or their insecurities?

Long before alternative therapies became popular my mother told us about one therapy she had tried. **Applied Kinesiology**. The practitioner found she was sensitive to a range of foods. To eliminate them from her diet required two separate menus. My step-father wasn't happy. Money was tight back then. He was unaware of the importance of nutrition and was definitely 'Old School'. He complained and complained, until she abandoned her effort. Later, when she became very sick, he realized he might lose her and became wonderfully devoted. Unfortunately, the damage was done.

What about you? If you are trying to heal, do you have support? Someone who may have gone through it themselves and knows what is involved? A fellow sufferer, perhaps?

Don't discount the Church. Spiritual power can 'move mountains' and the Christian, Muslim or Buddhist family are the largest in the world. You do not have to be a believer for them to welcome and support you.

Find a 'buddy' or contact Health Coaches like me. Contact me, online. If you need more structured support, try a retreat. There is no need to be alone and isolated. Stress, depression and anxiety can drive us into isolation, sometimes to the point we will not leave our homes. Do not succumb to this. Realize that, while most of us are preoccupied with our own problems, there are still good people out there who can help, even if only to listen. Be strong and keep your eye on the prize! Once others see you succeed they will no longer look at you as a burden but an inspiration.

Do not neglect this very important aspect of getting well. Good support can be the difference between success and failure.

"Mum Doesn't Look so Good"

Ellie was 70. Alzheimer's had taken hold and her family wanted to cure her. Or at least halt its progression. Her step-daughter signed up for a 3-day juice fast and was asking questions throughout. This was unusual. A few days after she completed the fast, I received a call.

"What shall I do? Mum doesn't look so good".

"Your mother? She is doing the program?" I asked, alarmed.

I rushed over to their hotel, to find her mother lying on the sofa, cold and listless.

"No. No. No!" I admonished. *"She is too frail to be fasting. Make her some warm, nourishing soup. Now!"*

The reason for all the questioning became clear. In order to save money, the daughter had signed up to a detox program and was feeding back how to do it, to the rest of her family. This is where a little bit of knowledge can be dangerous. She had pumped me for information, soaking up everything I taught her, but the crucial question of whether her mother should fast at all, never arose. Some constitutional types should NOT fast. If they are emaciated, they need building up, not depleting further. Strengthen first and then try. Or, better yet, adopt a gentler program. When it comes to health, there is more than one way to skin a cat

Fasting is perhaps the wrong label. Anyone juicing, is getting concentrated doses of vitamins and minerals, in liquid form. Far more than they could extract by chewing. When the digestive 'fire' is weak, nutrients in liquids are assimilated quickly. The body does not have to expend vital energy in digesting heavier, solid foods. More energy is freed to repair and heal. This idea that our 'vital force' is used for healing is called 'Vitalism'.

Caution must be exercised by anyone who is considering fasting. Your channels of elimination, lungs, liver, kidneys, colon and skin, must be working optimally **before** undertaking a detoxification program. You can become quite sick if you suddenly release a flood of toxins into your system. Experienced practitioners know what to do in such circumstances. The inexperienced do not.

Thankfully, poor Ellie recovered.

Are You Weak or Strong?

For many years Dr Richard Schulze took on those hospitals had sent home to die, and cured them. He was firm. If patients were not prepared to do as instructed he would not take them on.

Dr Dean Ornish has a heart program that restores the integrity of your cardiovascular system in 12-18 months. He is similarly firm. If you do not stick to the program, you are out.

Many of us experience an infant-like helplessness where we feel alone, isolated, weak and slaves to our addictions. Whether the internet, junk food, red wine, sticky buns, coffee or cigarettes, we don't believe we are capable of lifestyle changes and, let's be honest, don't WANT to change. When someone says we must, we become agitated and resentful. This is the nature of addiction. The person in front of you is telling you to give up your 'treats'. The means you use to self-tranquillize. Don't they know how dependent you are? Where are you going to get your 'fix' if you are forced to stop? Our cravings are powerful. Just the thought of stopping weakens our resolve. Our inner voice whispers, "I can't do it". Like New Year Resolutions, our determination to make healthy changes, lasts about 5 minutes even when, at an intellectual level, we know we are killing ourselves.

Even when things start to go well, we self-sabotage. Returning us to our uncomfortable 'comfort zone' or thrashing worn-out adrenals into life.

People love the information I share about diet, exercise, herbs, emotional healing and so on. They have never heard this knowledge explained with the kind of clarity I provide. They can't believe it is so simple. They are delighted to find someone to cut through the confusion. Then it hits them. They will have to make sacrifices. I can tell the ones that will fail. Usually with such people I apologize, tell them I cannot help them and ease them out the door. Unlike Harry Potter, I'm not a magician. If you aren't serious about being cured, why waste other's time? Practitioners, like Schulze and Ornish, do not need an undeserved reputation for failure by taking on those who lack motivation. Better to stay with a mainstream Doctor who is willing to give you what you want.

Staying on course sometimes requires a carrot and sometimes a stick. When I did my military service, heaven help you if you were a slacker. They soon licked you into shape. On one occasion I went through a two-week Royal Marine leadership course. The emphasis was on physical exercise and boy, did they put me through the wringer.

When I came out the other side, there was no way I could sit at home and be a couch potato. I HAD to go out and run, I was bursting with so much energy. Now I am 60 it is different. You cannot expect seniors with arthritic joints, heart disease or in a wheelchair, to start running up mountains, pounding pavements, being barked at by sadistic, shaven-headed Marines. There are less violent ways to get blood and lymph moving. Yet, there is a lesson here. If you are prepared to make the effort, even if starting with baby steps, your transformation will amaze you!

If you are feeling helpless and hopeless and struggling to stay on the healing path, DO NOT BE DISCOURAGED. **Doubt is a dragon we all have to slay**. As an addictive personality, I have had to slay many dragons over the years. When you see someone turned around from helplessness to hope, as often as I have, there is something magical about it. Strength and success lie within each of us.

Yes. I am talking about YOU. You are stronger than you think.

Peter Seeks the Easy Way

When bar owner Peter came to see me he could barely squeeze out of his car. Aged 54, grossly overweight, he had been burning the candle at both ends for too many years and was now paying the price. Peter had serious health problems and was on multiple medications. One step away from a coffin, Peter wanted to live a little longer.

"Wow. What a mess".

"Don't I know it", said Peter.

"How serious are you about getting healthy?"

"Very. I want a few more years with my daughters".

That was good enough for me.

"Ok", I said. *"You cannot do this the quick way. You have to do this slowly."*

What did I mean? Peter's body was 'filthy' from years of alcohol abuse, heavy smoking, no exercise, too many late nights and a diet of nutritionally-deficient, junk food. I doubt he had eaten a fresh vegetable in years. Almost certainly his channels of elimination were congested. Constipation, fatty liver, enlarged prostate, fluid retention, psoriasis, high blood pressure, poor circulation, body odour, Statins (and other risky medicines), acidosis. Add parasites and fungal infection. Putting Peter on a juice fast would release a flood of toxins into his bloodstream, driving up his blood pressure and overwhelming his liver and kidneys. Peter could die. Before he undertook a program, Peter needed to ensure his elimination channels were functioning optimally. I explained how he could do this. After listening, Peter was keen and hopeful. However, once he got home, he talked himself out of taking any action, wanting an easier way. Three months later Peter was dead. There wasn't an easier way.

Chapter 34
You Cannot Heal a Dirty Body

By now you will have understood, in natural healing there are two main causes of disease. Toxicity and deficiency. In order to heal, you must:

1. Remove toxins (clean the body).
2. Provide adequate nutrition.

Why does the body need to be clean? According to cancer specialists, Max and Charlotte Gerson, as well as the great healers, *"You cannot heal a dirty body"*.

There are several techniques for cleaning the body (detox). The most common are physical exercises, breathwork, steam sauna and massage, dry skin brushing, cleansing juices, raw vegetables, hydration, contrast bathing, liver and kidney flushes and bowel cleansing. Let's look at them, briefly.

Physical exercise gets the blood and lymph moving and opens up the pores, excreting toxins through the skin.

Breathing exercises. The body is flooded with oxygen and 'prana', revitalizing oxygen-starved cells and expelling waste gases.

Herbal steam saunas open the pores and raise body temperature. High temperatures kill off pathogens and liquefy solidified waste.

Massage helps release and mobilize toxins and move them toward the elimination channels.

Dry skin brushing removes dead skin layers, moves the blood and invigorates.

Juices and clean water, hydrate, cleanse and nourish our cells.

Contrast bathing is one of the best ways to get the blood circulating. Repeatedly switching between hot and cold water, will at first bring fresh blood to the surface of your skin, then drive it deeper. The improved circulation helps deliver healing herbs or nutrients to where they are needed.

Bowel cleansing Constipation, putrefaction, stagnation and fermentation encourage parasitic invasion and auto-intoxication (self-poisoning). Bowel pockets (diverticulitis) can cause inflammation, cramping, bloating and diarrhoea. Unbalanced gut bacteria (dysbiosis) needs to be corrected.

Liver, gall bladder and Kidney flushes help eliminate backed-up toxins. With the chemical/fungal assault we are under, our lymphatic (waste-disposal system) becomes backed-up with waste. The liver and kidneys need to be looked after.

Some cleansing programs are gentle and some aggressive. For instance, you can encourage elimination of waste with gentle laxative teas or uniodized sea salt. Castor oil, Epsom salts or enemas are also effective at moving the bowels. More aggressively, on the 'Master Cleanse', you drink 2 litres of salt water, in under 40 minutes, which flushes the bowels rapidly. An advanced Yoga cleansing method I undertake is to drink warm, salt water, two glasses at a time, followed by five different stretching exercises, until you have drunk 32 glasses. This forces salt water into every nook and cranny of the colon. This 6-monthly routine takes around three hours and is not just a cleanse but a workout!

Ayurveda has an excellent cleansing protocol, called 'Panchakarma', which uses heat, therapeutic massage, warm oil treatments and enemas, to liquefy and mobilize toxins and excrete them.

The word 'Detox' is plastered on just about every product these days. Care needs to be exercised with regard to quality. e.g. You don't want to be taking in chemicals used to bleach your 'detox' herbal tea bags.

Some sceptics will tell you toxins do not exist. They are convinced the liver detoxifies everything and if it didn't, we would be poisoned or dead. Such people are being too literal and their knowledge is out of date. The U.S. CDC (Centre for Disease Control) has identified hundreds of chemicals found in human and breast tissue and published the fact. Worried mothers have turned away from breast-feeding, to infant formula, out of concern. Except infant formula is also contaminated and lacks the protection breast milk provides. Breast-feeding is still the best way to nourish and protect the new-born.

Unborn children are at serious risk from at least 12 developmental neurotoxins we know of and more we do not. According to researchers, **a 'silent pandemic' of chemical contamination is occurring on a global scale**.

Chemicals like DDT, BPA (from plastics). Poisons, like arsenic and fluoride. Heavy metals like mercury, lead and aluminium.

Parasites; fungi; bacteria; by-products of poor digestion; acid wastes; 'electrosmog' (radiation from mobile phones, computers, electrical devices and nuclear testing); even recreational and pharmaceutical drug residues.

In a healthy person, these should be mopped up efficiently and excreted. In someone whose health is compromised, they can accumulate and be stored in body tissue. Some studies show even the fit have 500 different chemicals detectable in the body.

Sceptical minds do not understand when we talk about detox. Remember the 5 Layers? Physical toxins are not the only toxins. We have toxic thoughts, toxic emotions and toxic relationships. The word 'detox' encompasses them all.

Hydration is crucial. Think of a dirty sponge. If you place a dirty sponge in a bucket of cold water and leave it overnight, the next morning the sponge is clean and the dirt is laying on the bottom of the bucket. Same principle with us. Ordinarily we should be taking in enough clean water, via drinking and from fruits and vegetables, to allow proper hydration and elimination. However, most of us are not taking in sufficient fluids and are dehydrated. Contaminants and metabolic waste products are thus not mobilized and expelled and find their way to the small capillaries, such as in our joints, where they lodge, causing inflammation and degeneration. During a detox, we flood our tissues with fluids, then use manipulation (massage) and agitation (exercise), to mobilize and move waste to the channels of elimination. This is why cleansing programs like the **Gerson Therapy** or the **Master Cleanse** (Lemonade Diet) require you to drink fluid every hour, throughout the day.

Many massage therapists are really only 'oil-smearers'. This is inadequate. You need muscles, nerves, lymph nodes and tissues to be kneaded and pressed. When I go for a Thai Traditional massage, the masseuse asks if I would like soft, medium or strong pressure?

"None", I say. "Give me a savage beating".

I am only half-joking. I want FIRM pressure. As much as I can tolerate. I am not there to relax but to clear congestion and improve circulation. If you cannot find affordable, effective massage, have friends or family do it. We all know instinctively what to do. Who doesn't love a head massage? TRY. Your Doctor certainly isn't going to put his hands on you.

"The soil is our external metabolism. It must be free of herbicides and pesticides or the body cannot heal."
- Dr. Max Gerson

Chapter 35
Look in the Mirror

When a villager with a smile that can light up the sky says, *"foreigners think too much"*, it is a reminder of how much the West has given primacy to the mind.

There is much to be learned from other peoples. In my travels to more than 50 countries, I have lived amongst Chinese, Thais, Portuguese, Indians, Russians, Arabs and more. With few exceptions, the local people met me with brilliant, friendly smiles. The exceptions? Well, when showing Russian friends photographs, one asked "Why are you showing your teeth?" In Moscow and St. Petersburg I rarely saw anyone smile in the street, yet experienced genuine warmth inside Russian homes. They are also amused by my beach pictures. "Why do you want your skin brown?" White-skinned western populations equate tanned skin with health. Brown-skinned populations equate white skin with success. The latter avoid the sun and damage their skin with harsh bleaching chemicals to try to be whiter. The former seek out the sun and damage their skin with harsh suntan lotions to try to be browner. The media and advertising world encourage both behaviours, to shift product. The result? Millions unhappy with their appearance.

What do you see when you look in the mirror? Are you aware how much your perception of yourself has been shaped by corporations? The goal of the Merchant Class is to make us dissatisfied with who we are and what we have, in order to sell solutions. They create markets, in order to service them. Be it cosmetics, 'diet' products, suntan lotion or sneakers. Liberating yourself from this brainwashing is crucial if you wish to be self-confident and free.

For all its faults, religion has a better model. We are perfect in God's eyes, made 'in the image of God'. Not convinced, by an advertising company, we are too fat, too white, too black, our teeth too yellow or misshapen, nose too big and breasts too small.

As a health advocate I feel pressure to look young for my age, vibrantly healthy and athletic. That's what people expect. To them, it shows I don't just 'talk the talk' but also 'walk the walk'. I am not sure why. Most Doctors look unhealthy yet still practice. I once suggested to an artist friend I might have a little 'nip and tuck'. Remove the skin under my eyes and from around my neck which, in my advancing years, looks rather like that of a freshly plucked chicken. Unacceptable, in this 'anti-aging' culture. To her credit, my artist friend said,

"If you change a thing, I'll kill you!"

Artists are excited by character, not conformity. I knew she was right, so accepted my outer coating isn't going to get any younger, and my life experiences, good or bad, will remain etched permanently onto my face. If you have read my blog post **'Don't Call Me "Guru"'** (<u>19</u>) you know I reject pressure which pushes you to be something you are not.

Here's my rather base suggestion. Stick two fingers up at the marketing manipulators and STAND TALL. LOVE yourself, every single part of you. What kind of a boring world would it be if we all looked like Brad Pitt and Angelina Jolie?

Coming back to smiling. In India, Cambodia, Laos, Vietnam and Thailand, the villagers smiled instantly and would invite me in for 'chai' (tea), or food. In India, this impressed me so much I decided to conduct an experiment. For a two week period I would smile at every traveller I met. The result was revealing. European and American travellers were universally stone-faced when approaching each other. Many would not look me in the eye. They seemed pre-occupied, troubled and somewhat alarmed when I smiled at them. Why is this weird man grinning at me? A few returned the smile, in surprise and pleasure.

We have forgotten how to smile at each other. To relax and greet each other as fellow inhabitants of this beautiful planet. To experience the joy of new encounters and new friends. There is a fascinating video, online, showing laughter being deliberately provoked, on a New York subway train. One man with an infectious laugh started it. Before long, everyone was laughing. Try it next time you are out and about. Or if you can't bring yourself to chuckle, smile at everyone you meet and see the reaction you get. Call it **'The Great Smile Challenge'**. You will make someone's day, just as the villagers made mine.

"It's Only Two a Day!"

I could hear the gasping of the over-laden 'tuk-tuk' (motorbike taxi) as it climbed the hill and pulled up in front of the gate. From my rear garden, I watched three ladies disembark. Dawn, young and heavy. Susan, middle aged, her desire to stay attractive evidenced by too much rouge and silicone-enhanced breasts. Erin, elderly and obese, so much so she struggled to climb out of the vehicle. These ladies had heard of me and wished to discuss their various health issues.

Dawn had been an exceptional athlete, representing her country in gymnastics, until a family tragedy triggered over-eating, weight gain, deep depression and constant exhaustion. For 12 years Doctors and psychiatrists had been unable to figure out what was wrong with her. Dawn was tired of being drugged and depressed.

Susan was different. She didn't look ill. Unless trying to stay young is a disease. No. Susan was on a mission to help her sick mother, suffering from Alzheimer's.

Erin was seriously unwell. Cancer, heart disease, obesity and more. She had spent years in and out of hospitals, undergoing multiple operations.

Drinks were served, pleasantries exchanged and I started to share my knowledge. It quickly became apparent Erin was clued-up on alternative medicine. There was little she didn't know and hadn't tried. She became excited as I spoke, constantly confirming my statements and offering some of her own. I mentioned the importance of cleansing. She told us about her detox. I moved onto useful local herbs. She brought up American equivalents. I covered nutrition. She related the diets she had tried. It was all hugely supportive. The meeting was going swimmingly, until Erin reached into her bag, pulled out a cigarette and lit up.

"Gasp!"

We were shocked. How on earth can a person who is seriously ill, with tremendous knowledge of how to get well, still smoke? There was a huge contradiction at work. I explained to Erin I could not help her if she smoked.

"But it's only two a day!" she cried.

"I'm sorry. Those are my rules".

That was the last I saw of Erin.

Chapter 36
What You Have Learned?

Well, here we are, at the end of our journey together. I hope this personal view, of what is a vast subject, health, has been of some help.

My aim in writing the book was to:

1. Guide you toward better health.
2. Explain why mainstream medicine will never cure.
3. Shed light on why Alternative medicine also fails to cure, unless you have the right tools in your healing toolbox and apply them appropriately. You cannot take a water-pistol to an inferno.
4. Have you understand, no matter how low you feel, or desperate your situation, there is always hope. NEVER let any puffed-up 'expert' or authority-figure take hope away from you.
5. Point out, experts are rarely right. Trust your own instincts.
6. Educate you in how to heal yourself, rather than rely on those who do not have an answer and know nothing about you.
7. Have you focus on the RIGHT way to reverse disease and not waste time, energy and money on the WRONG.
8. Encourage you to reclaim power over what you are putting into your mouth and have you consider whether what you are eating and drinking is building health or disease? The apple or the doughnut.
9. Inspire you to free yourself from addiction, using tools like juice-fasting, the 'Bitter' taste, EFT and 'Breaking the Chains'
10. Show you how to dissolve toxic emotions that drive you to self-tranquillize.
11. Show you healing is NOT complicated. We just make it that way.
12. Have you understand, at a deeper level, you are a wonderful creation, whose body really is a Temple. That, no matter how poor your external environment, you can be the Lotus Flower.
13. Put you in touch with your inner SELF. The shining light, that makes you fully human. That aspect you have neglected for so long.
14. Encourage you to stick with ONE program and not bounce from therapy to therapy.

15. Have you question over-medicalization and whether you need… or can rely on… all those tests.
16. Help you understand you are not healing a specific disorder but strengthening the body and giving it everything it needs to heal, so ALL your disorders will resolve.
17. Show you natural healing does not dependent on diagnosis.
18. Introduce you to forgotten healing knowledge.
19. Remind you the **Laws of Nature** always bring consequences when violated.
20. Remind you that, while violating Nature's Laws can **cause** disease, living in accordance with them can **prevent** and **reverse** it.
21. Have you take action NOW and not wait and wait until your disease is so far gone it becomes more difficult to resolve, or you are dead.
22. Have you realise your health is **priceless**. Invest in it!
23. Let you know you need not do this alone. Support is out there. *'Seek and ye shall find'*.

The Next Step

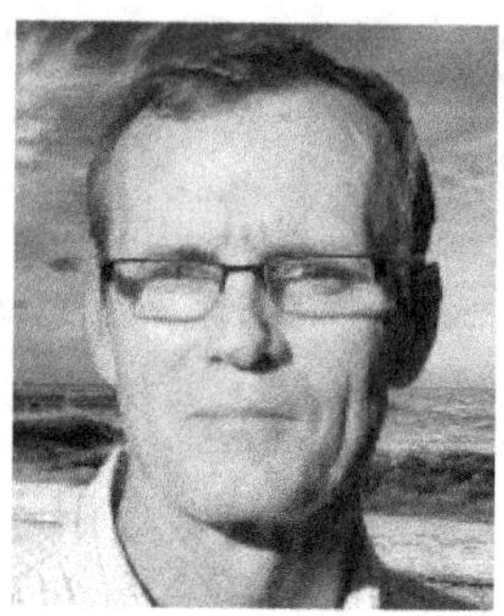

Well done! I have done my bit. Now it is your turn. To put into action what you have learned in these pages. To resist moving on to the next book, guru, TV Doctor, or friend who says they have a better way.

Remember why you are doing this…

"We all deserve a life of glowing health and vitality, free from pain and sickness, whether in Body, Mind or Spirit. It is our birthright. To be happy. To be at peace. To enjoy a long, healthy existence on this beautiful planet. To love ourselves, our families and our fellow man and to pass away peacefully in our sleep."

Worth striving for, don't you think? Do not stay unhappy and unhealthy a day longer. Take a vow right now.

"Today, I make a promise. I am going to get better. Nothing is going to get in my way. I am a unique and beautiful child of God (or Nature). No longer will I allow those who care nothing for me, to destroy my health. I am taking back my life. When I experience moments of weakness, I will not crumble. Instead I will use such moments to strengthen my resolve."

Memorize it. Make a poster and put it on your wall. Repeat this and other affirmations **every day**. Well done. Now just do it. And when you have done it, let me know via my website, Facebook or email, how you are getting on. If you feel you are struggling or cannot do it alone, by all means contact me at paulkeenan@antarana.com and let's see what miracles can be achieved.

"Wishing you the very **BEST** of health!" - **Paul**

Appendix

What are Doshas?

The Doshas are a set of characteristics in India's Ayurvedic medicine, similar to the ancient Greek concept of "humours," which were unfortunately misused (and hence given a bad press) in the West. The three doshas: **Vata** (Air), **Pitta** (Fire) and **Kapha** (Earth or Water) are used to describe people based on their physical, mental, emotional and psychological characteristics. Each dosha reflects one or more of the base elements. Earth, Air, Fire and Water.

The Meaning of a "Dosha"

Ayurvedic traditions recognize and honour the uniqueness of each individual, but the highest virtue is balance. It is believed every person requires different ingredients for optimal health, to balance their doshas and their particular constitutional type. Ayurveda means "The Science (or Knowledge) of Life," while Dosha means each of three energies believed to circulate in the body and govern physiological activity. Every person possesses some of the qualities of all three doshas. The unique balance between Air, Fire, Earth & Water (Vata, Pitta, Kapha) determines a person's constitution, body type, and mental and emotional strengths and weaknesses.

Finding Your Dosha Type

Most people will have one predominant dosha, but others have two or all three in equal balance. Dozens of tests and resources are available online to help identify your Dosha.

The Three Doshas

Vata (Air)

Vata dosha is composed of the elements of air and space (or ether). Vata is dry, cool, light, clear and active. It governs breathing, elimination, motor skills and the senses.

People who have a Vata constitution are noticeably tall or short, with a light frame, small musculature, and low body fat. They usually have dry hair and skin, low body temperature and blood pressure, a small mouth and grey, brown or blue eyes.

Vata temperament is quick and clever, but impatient and lacking in stamina. Vata people are commonly active and creative, but they tend to sleep lightly and may be shy, anxious and insecure.

Vata imbalance can cause worries, insomnia, fluctuating appetite, cramps and constipation. Vata governs the other two doshas and is usually the first cause of illness or disease.

Foods that are warm, moist, mildly spicy and well-cooked, balance and contain Vata.

Pitta (Fire)

Pitta is predominantly fire with some water. It is hot, light, liquid, sour, sharp and oily. Pitta governs metabolism and digestive processes of the mind, body and spirit; intelligence and understanding; hunger and thirst; and the fiery emotions of anger, hate and jealousy.

Pitta people are of medium build, with fair skin that may show freckles or blemishes, a medium-sized mouth, and blue or hazel eyes.

Those with pitta temperament are organized, ambitious and driven but easily irritated. They love knowledge and possess leadership abilities. Although they are competitive, controlling and judgmental, they usually accomplish a great deal. They have strong digestive systems, moderate stamina and enjoy physical activity.

Pitta governs the small intestine, stomach, skin, eyes, fat, sweat and blood. Imbalance often shows as impatience, hostility, and emotional outbursts which can affect these physical areas.

Pitta should avoid cigarettes and anything heating or aggravating to the body's systems. Foods to soothe pitta are cool, sweet, bitter and astringent.

Kapha (Earth/Water)

Kapha combines the elements of 'Water' and 'Earth', and has the most physicality of the three doshas. Kapha is cool, heavy, dense, slow, and liquid, and governs the joints, strength, the heart, lungs and wound healing.

Kapha people are usually heavier than other types due to slower metabolism, with cool or oily skin, dark eyes, large lips and thick, wavy hair. They are relaxed, patient, compassionate, and steady. They neither learn nor accept change easily, but they have steady energy and stamina. They may seem withdrawn or impassionate.

Excess Kapha results in emotional attachment and clinginess, greed, and envy. It can also contribute to weight gain, lethargy, congestion and allergies.

Foods with the opposite properties to earth and water, (i.e. cold, heavy and mucus-forming) are warm, light, dry, spicy and bitter and will balance Kapha. These types do well on vegan and vegetarian diets.

To learn more about Ayurveda, seek books by either David Frawley or Vasant Lad.

Sources

For your convenience, I have created a web page listing ALL the links in the book. To view, enter the following into your browser:
https://www.antarana.com/sources--fydcl.html

1. Contaminants in human milk: weighing the risks against the benefits of breastfeeding.
https://www.ncbi.nlm.nih.gov/pubmed/?term=PMC2569122

2. The Cochrane Collaboration
http://nordic.cochrane.org/

3. Dr Duke's Phytochemical and Ethnobotanical Database
https://phytochem.nal.usda.gov/phytochem/plants/show/942?et=

4. Impact of fluoride on neurological development in children
https://www.hsph.harvard.edu/news/features/fluoride-childrens-health-grandjean-choi/

5. Detection of Glyphosate Residues in Animals and Humans
http://omicsonline.org/open-access/detection-of-glyphosate-residues-in-animals-and-humans-2161-0525.1000210.pdf

6. Glyphosate, pathways to modern diseases II: Celiac sprue and gluten intolerance
http://www.ncbi.nlm.nih.gov/pmc/articles/PMC3945755/

7. Confessions of an Economic Hitman
https://www.youtube.com/watch?v=272uQ-MNUdQ

8. Nutrition and Health – The Association between Eating Behaviour and Various Health Parameters: A Matched Sample Study
https://www.ncbi.nlm.nih.gov/pmc/articles/PMC3917888/

9. How Healing Becomes a Crime
https://www.youtube.com/watch?v=JXNGBYQGOdw

10. Scientific Papers Linking Thimerosal Exposure to Autism

https://www.focusforhealth.org/wp-content/uploads/2015/03/Scientific-Papers-Showing-Linking-Thimerosal-Exposure-to-Autism-4-6-15.pdf

11. The Marvellous Health of Unvaccinated Children
http://www.vaccinationcouncil.org/2010/06/25/the-marvellous-health-of-unvaccinated-children/

12. Vitamin cartel companies given record fines
http://www.ncbi.nlm.nih.gov/pmc/articles/PMC1173053/

13. Nothing Boring About Boron
https://www.ncbi.nlm.nih.gov/pmc/articles/PMC4712861/

14. The Borax Conspiracy
http://www.health-science-spirit.com/borax.htm

15. Diet reverses Type 2 Diabetes
http://www.ncl.ac.uk/press/news/2015/10/type2diabetes/

16. Dr Schulze Intestinal Formula
https://www.herbdoc.com/intestinal-formula-2

17. Toxic Stress
https://developingchild.harvard.edu/science/key-concepts/toxic-stress/

18. Understanding nutrition, depression and mental illness
http://www.ncbi.nlm.nih.gov/pmc/articles/PMC2738337/

19. Don't Call Me "Guru"
https://www.antarana.com/health-blog/the-perils-of-being-a-guru

20. How Independent Are Vaccine Defenders?
https://www.cbsnews.com/news/how-independent-are-vaccine-defenders/

21. A new, evidence-based estimate of patient harms associated with hospital care. https://www.ncbi.nlm.nih.gov/pubmed/23860193

May I Ask a Favour?

Did you enjoy the book? If so, I could very much use your help to get it in front of others.

Here's how...

1. **WRITE A POSITIVE BOOK REVIEW**
   On Amazon or wherever you purchased it. (Hint... hint... do it now before you are distracted and forget.)

2. If you know someone struggling with their health, send them a copy as a gift, recommend, or send a <u>link to the book</u>.

3. If you use **social media**, 'Like', 'Share', 'Follow', discuss, recommend, bookmark, forward, chat, message or carrier pigeon.

4. If your health has improved using any of the protocols mentioned, please submit a testimonial. I would love to hear from you.

5. Do not let this be the end of our journey together. Follow me on Facebook or my blog.

Facebook
https://www.facebook.com/PaulKeenanAuthor/

Health Blog
https://www.antarana.com/health-blog

Retreats and Health Coaching

I am always happy to receive new and returning guests and chat to clients 'live'. Please review a sample of our offerings. If you do not see your condition, allow us to design a program for you! We have recently added a '**Candida Cleanse**', even an '**End Your Smartphone Addiction**' retreat!

Retreats
https://www.antarana.com/retreats.html

Consultations
https://www.antarana.com/coaching.html

Sample Programs

Healing Depression, Stress & Anxiety
Reverse Diabetes
Reversing Chronic Disease
Life After Cancer
Master Cleanse Detox
Fluoride Detox
Candida Cleanse
End Your Smartphone Addiction!

Contact Us

Email for further information: info@antarana.com

Giving Back

The following causes will receive income from sales of the book.

Power of Love Children's Home
Rescue Paws Animal sanctuary
Lem – A Thai villager with Stage IV Lung Cancer

Details on our **Giving Back** page.
https://www.antarana.com/giving-back.html

COMING SOON

FIRE YOUR PSYCHIATRIST!

by

Paul Keenan

The French were very good at separating the head from the body, with their Guillotine. Unsurprisingly, people did not find it a healing experience. So why does Psychiatry separate the head from the body and expect people to improve?

In a world where drugging of the masses has become normal, Paul Keenan uses straightforward language to drive a coach and horses through the nonsense being peddled by so-called mental health experts. 6 million children in the U.S. are being given Class II narcotics for behaviour that can be corrected by better parenting, proper nutrition, eliminating 'excito-toxic' chemicals, heavy metals and sugars, and reducing poverty. Millions of adults are given 'chemical coshes' because they are suffering toxic STRESS, caused by toxic politicians, toxic medicine, toxic media, toxic food and a toxic environment.

The consequences of swallowing poisonous fluoride compounds, otherwise known as anti-depressants, are addiction, suicide, impotence and permanent brain changes. For benefits which have been exaggerated. We truly are a Zombie Nation.

Natural and Alternatives remedies are unfairly vilified for not having evidence to support them. Yet, psychiatry has even less (has anyone ever seen a test for a 'chemical imbalance of the brain'?) yet is fully supported by government. 25% of Americans are diagnosed with a mental disorder. One quarter of the population. Are these people really 'mad' or is there something you aren't being told?